Atlas of Non-Invasive Imaging in Cardiac Anatomy

Francesco F. Faletra · Jagat Narula
Siew Yen Ho
Editors

Atlas of Non-Invasive Imaging in Cardiac Anatomy

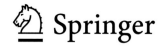 Springer

Editors
Francesco F. Faletra
Department of Cardiology
Cardiocentro Ticino
Lugano
Switzerland

Siew Yen Ho
Royal Brompton Hospital
London
UK

Jagat Narula
Icahn School of Medicine at Mount Sinai
New York, NY
USA

ISBN 978-3-030-35505-0   ISBN 978-3-030-35506-7   (eBook)
https://doi.org/10.1007/978-3-030-35506-7

This Springer imprint is published by the registered company Springer Nature Switzerland AG
The registered company address is: Gewerbestrasse 11, 6330 Cham, Switzerland

To my wife, Gratiela, for her love and patience.
To my staff for their encouragement.

Francesco F. Faletra

To two youngest members in my lovely family, my son – Sukrit,
and grandson – Arun.

Jagat Narula

Preface

Cardiac morphology is probably the most captivating branch of the discipline of anatomy. Indeed, the first description of cardiac anatomy can be found in the Ebers Papyrus from pre-Hippocratic era. The Egyptians considered the heart as the origin of all vessels and correlated vessel pulsatility to cardiac contractility. Subsequently, Hippocrates and his colleagues wrote the first book with detailed description of the anatomy of the heart and the cardiovascular system. In the Greek era, Herophilus distinguished arteries from veins based on their structure, and Erasistratus provided the description of heart valves. In the Roman era, Galen described the vena cava and hepatic veins connecting with the right ventricle through the right atrium and explicitly distinguished between inlet and outlet valves.

In the medieval era, Leonardo da Vinci made the most impressive contributions to cardiac anatomy; some of his imaginative descriptions and drawings amaze even the modern-day morphologists. He described four heart chambers, as we know them today, and distinguished the atria from the appendages. The most celebrated of his contributions was the study of the aortic root: his drawings of the aortic root, leaflets, and the vortex in the sinuses are among the most startling in the history of medicine.

In the sixteenth century, the University of Padua Medical School played a fundamental role in advancing the knowledge of cardiac anatomy. Andreas Vesalius, a famous teacher of Anatomy and Surgery, published two books entitled *Six Anatomical Tables* and *The Factory of the Human Body* highlighting the left atrioventricular valve as the *mitral valve* because of its resemblance with a bishop's miter. In the seventeenth century, other eminent anatomists including Colombo, Harvey, Lower, and Stensen refined the anatomic structure of the heart as a four-chambered organ and the passage of blood through the heart, lungs, and the entire body. Vieussens, Thebesius, de Senac, and Scarpa continued to explore in the next century and defined the anatomy of coronary arteries, cardiac veins, coronary sinus, Thebesian valve, and mitral subvalvular apparatus.

Hundreds of publications have since then been written by cardiac anatomists who have extensively reported the morphological and functional characteristics of the heart. However, these publications have seldom reached the cardiology community, and the clinical cardiologists have remained oblivious to the anatomical research. For centuries, the anatomy of heart has been taught to the medical students in the dissection halls using cadavers, with limited understanding of three-dimensional orientation of the complex organ.

In the past two decades, sophisticated imaging techniques, such as computed tomography, cardiac magnetic resonance imaging, and three-dimensional echocardiography, have been able to illustrate anatomical details of the heart with a previously unimaginable quality. These diagnostic techniques have predominantly been used only for diagnostic purposes. However, these imaging modalities can provide an enormous source of high spatial and temporal resolution compared with normal macroscopic images of cardiac structures and can offer most valuable aids for teaching anatomy to medical students. Because of their *three-dimensional* nature, every cardiac structure can be seen in countless perspectives.

The main objective of this atlas is to compare and contrast the sophisticated anatomical silhouettes with the exquisite imaging details. In particular, this book will focus on the anatomic structures which are most relevant for clinical cardiologists and cardiac interventionalists.

To document the actual anatomy with fidelity, most noninvasive images are accompanied side by side with anatomical specimens.

We are convinced that in the third millennium medical students and, in particular, cardiologists will be able to learn cardiac anatomy through *in vivo* imaging. This must become the preferred mode of teaching in medical schools as an additional tool to the classic anatomy through cadaveric dissection and anatomic specimens. We sincerely hope that this book will help the evolution of cardiologists who will be adept with bedside imaging and rapid diagnostic algorithms.

Lugano, Switzerland   Francesco F. Faletra
London, UK   Siew Yen Ho
New York, NY, USA   Jagat Narula

Contents

Contributors

Marco Araco, MD Interventional Cardiology Department, Fondazione Cardiocentro Ticino, Lugano, Switzerland

Tiziano Cassina, PhD, MD Cardiac Anesthesiology and Intensive Care Unit, Fondazione Cardiocentro Ticino, Lugano, Switzerland

Stefanos Demertzis, PhD, MD Cardiac Surgery Department, Fondazione Cardiocentro Ticino, Lugano, Switzerland

Francesco F. Faletra, MD Non-invasive Cardiovascular Imaging Department, Fondazione Cardiocentro Ticino, Lugano, Switzerland

Enrico Ferrari, PhD, MD Cardiac Surgery Department, Fondazione Cardiocentro Ticino, Lugano, Switzerland

Siew Yen Ho, PhD Royal Brompton Hospital, Sydney Street, London, UK

Laura A. Leo, MD Non-invasive Cardiovascular Imaging Department, Fondazione Cardiocentro Ticino, Lugano, Switzerland

Marco Moccetti, MD Interventional Cardiology Department, Fondazione Cardiocentro Ticino, Lugano, Switzerland

Tiziano Moccetti, PhD, MD Cardiology Department, Fondazione Cardiocentro Ticino, Lugano, Switzerland

Jagat Narula, MD, PhD Icahn School of Medicine at Mount Sinai, New York, NY, USA

Vera L. Paiocchi, MD Non-invasive Cardiovascular Imaging Department, Fondazione Cardiocentro Ticino, Lugano, Switzerland

Elena Pasotti, MD Cardiology Department, Fondazione Cardiocentro Ticino, Lugano, Switzerland

Giovanni Pedrazzini, PhD, MD Cardiology Department, Fondazione Cardiocentro Ticino, Lugano, Switzerland

Susanne A. Schlossbauer, MD Non-invasive Cardiovascular Imaging Department, Fondazione Cardiocentro Ticino, Lugano, Switzerland

The Mitral Valve

Francesco F. Faletra, Tiziano Cassina, Laura A. Leo,
Vera L. Paiocchi, Siew Yen Ho, and Jagat Narula

In 1972, David E. Perloff, a cardiologist, and William Roberts, an anatomist, wrote the most educational paper on the mitral valve. These authors clarified that the mitral valve is not merely a couple of connective tissue flaps closing and opening secondary to the pressure gradient; it is a much more complex apparatus formed by several components working together in synchrony. Indeed, a perfect systolic competence of the valve and an unrestricted inflow requires precise spatial and temporal coordination. Only a reciprocal interaction between all the components will enable the normal function of the valve as a whole. Any anatomic change or disruption of one or more components inevitably causes mitral regurgitation. Anatomically, the valve consists of the mitral annulus, anterior and posterior leaflets, and the subvalvular apparatus of the chordae tendineae and papillary muscles. Because each of these components has a specific function, we will discuss them individually.

Mitral Annulus

In the cardiology community, the *mitral annulus* is commonly perceived as a circular ring of dense connective tissue from which the leaflets are suspended. The real architecture of the mitral annulus is different from this "traditional" description, and in many aspects the mitral annulus is just a *concept* rather than a well-defined anatomic entity. Moreover, anatomists, surgeons, imagers, and others have used terms such as *atrio-ventricular orifice*, *atrio-ventricular plane*, *valve hinge*, and *mitral hinge line* to describe the same structure, causing confusion. The aim of this chapter therefore is to provide a clear description of this essential component of the mitral valve complex. For simplicity, we will continue to name this part of the valve the *annulus*. The posterior and anterior segments of the mitral annulus differ in structure and function, so they are described separately.

The Posterior Annulus

The posterior annulus, longer than its anterior partner, suspends the posterior leaflet and can be portrayed roughly as a letter "C" extending posteriorly from the left to the right trigones.

From an anatomical point of view, it can be described as the convergence of three structures: the atrial wall, the leaflet hinge, and the marginal free wall of the left ventricle. These structures are thought to be connected by a discrete band of fibrous tissue, giving the impression of a solid annulus (Fig. 1.1a). In reality, however, the fibrous band often is discontinuous, and when present, may have different consistency and robustness. There are differences in thickness and density not only among different individuals but also along different segments of the same annulus. In those parts in which the fibrous band is absent, the posterior leaflet is inserted directly on the ventricular myocardium. Because of this anatomical arrangement, the posterior annulus follows the myocardial contraction and relaxation, playing a fundamental role in the sphincter action (Fig. 1.1b).

From a surgeon's viewpoint (that is, viewing from the left atrial side), this fibrous band is not visible. When present, it is located 2–3 mm external to the hinge line of the leaflet. What

F. F. Faletra (✉) · L. A. Leo · V. L. Paiocchi
Non-invasive Cardiovascular Imaging Department, Fondazione
Cardiocentro Ticino, Lugano, Switzerland
e-mail: Francesco.Faletra@cardiocentro.org;
lauraanna.leo@cardiocentro.org; vera.paiocchi@cardiocentro.org

T. Cassina
Cardiac Anesthesiology and Intensive Care Unit, Fondazione
Cardiocentro Ticino, Lugano, Switzerland
e-mail: tiziano.cassina@cardiocentro.org

S. Y. Ho
Royal Brompton Hospital, Sydney Street, London, UK
e-mail: yen.ho@imperial.ac.uk

J. Narula
Icahn School of Medicine at Mount Sinai, New York, NY, USA
e-mail: narula@mountsinai.org

© Springer Nature Switzerland AG 2020
F. F. Faletra et al. (eds.), *Atlas of Non-Invasive Imaging in Cardiac Anatomy*, https://doi.org/10.1007/978-3-030-35506-7_1

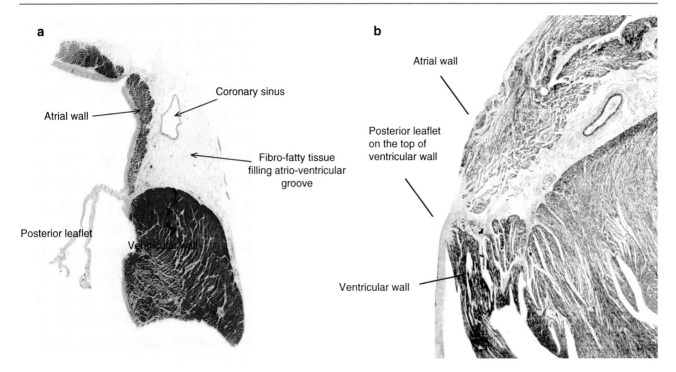

Fig. 1.1 (a) Histologic section of normal mitral valve stained in Massons trichrome stain showing fibrous tissue in green and myocardium in red. Note the fibrofatty tissue plane separating atrial from ventricular myocardium. (b) Histologic section of another normal mitral valve shows a less well-formed 'annulus'. Trichrome stain colors fibrous tissue green and myocardium in red. The posterior leaflet is inserted directly on the top of ventricular wall and has fibrous extensions into the atrial wall and atrioventricular groove

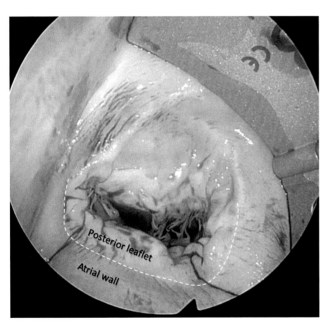

Fig. 1.2 Surgical view of the mitral valve. The *dotted line* marks the transition zone between the atrial wall and the posterior leaflet

the surgeons are clearly able to see is the "transition zone" between the atrial wall and the leaflet—the so-called *atrio-valvular junction* (Fig. 1.2).

Finally, *from an imager's point of view*, the cross sections obtained by computed tomography (CT), cardiac magnetic resonance (CMR), transthoracic echocardiography (TTE), and transesophageal echocardiography (TEE) show the line of insertion of the posterior leaflet (hinge line). This line is the fulcrum upon which the leaflet opens and closes during the cardiac cycle. The CT scan is the best imaging modality to clarify the anatomy of this region. The spatial resolution of this technique, with the voxel as small as 0.6 mm, allows precise definition of the anatomy of the region. Different slices show the extreme variability of the anatomical relationship between the hinge line of the posterior leaflet and the vessels lying in the atrioventricular groove, reflecting the changeable relationships of the vessels as they course through the fat-filled groove (Fig. 1.3).

On the other hand, the unique ability of cine sequences of CMR to obtain strong signals from both blood and fat, coupling with weak signal from myocardium, provides images

Fig. 1.3 CT images showing cross sections of the posterior annulus in the four-chamber view (**a**), two-chamber view (**c**), and long-axis view (**e**). Magnified images of the areas in the red squares are shown in panels (**b**), (**d**), and (**f**), respectively. The variable spatial relationship between fat, leaflet hinge, myocardium, and vessels is evident. *Cx* circumflex artery, *CS* coronary sinus, *LAA* left atrial appendage, *MB* marginal branch

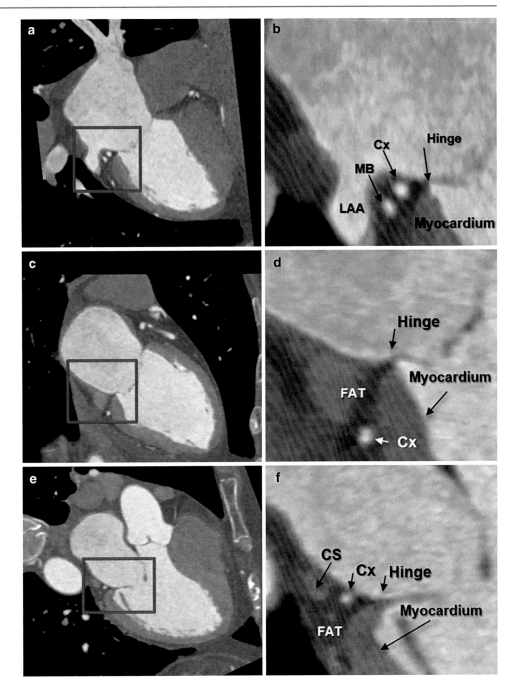

that reveal the adipose tissue that envelops the coronary arteries in the atrioventricular groove. This tissue contributes to the electrical insulation between left atrium and ventricle. Moreover, its presence is supposed to provide mechanical protection of the coronary arteries, buffering them against the torsion induced by the arterial pulse wave and cardiac contraction (Fig. 1.4).

TTE and TEE cross sections parallel images of CT and CMR, but the spatial resolution of the 2D TTE and TEE images is inferior to CT, and the tissue differentiation (differentiating fat from muscle) is less than with CMR because of the minimal differences in acoustic impedance between these two tissues. On the other hand, 3D TEE from an overhead perspective (surgical view) shows unique images of the

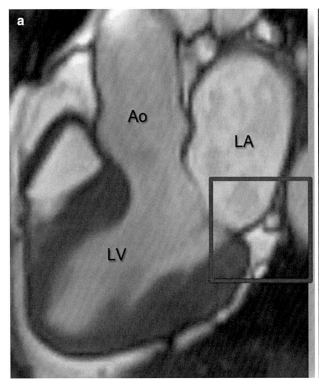 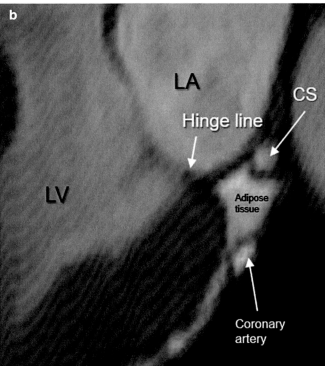

Fig. 1.4 (a) Cardiac magnetic resonance (CMR) cine images in long-axis view, obtained with steady-state free precession (SSFP). (b) The magnified image (*red square*) shows the atrioventricular groove with high-signal fat accumulation and vessels. The muscular tissue has a low signal and is easily distinguishable from blood and fat. The coronary sinus (CS) is often located in a more atrial position with respect to the atrioventricular groove. *Ao* aorta, *LA* left atrium, *LV* left ventricle

"sphincteric" action of the annulus (Fig. 1.5). Still, neither CT, CMR, or TTE and TEE are capable of detecting the fibrous band as a distinct structure.

Two vessels are usually close to the posterior mitral annulus: the circumflex artery and the great cardiac vein continuing into the coronary sinus. The circumflex artery runs between the base of the left atrial appendage and the anterior-lateral commissure, initially a few millimeters from the hinge of the posterior leaflet; it then moves away from the posterior annulus. The great cardiac vein continuing into the coronary sinus borders the attachment of the posterior leaflet laterally, posteriorly, and then medially, opening in the right atrium just close to the medial commissure. The relationship between the hinge line of the posterior mitral leaflet and the coronary sinus is of particular relevance because of the potential percutaneous treatment of functional mitral regurgitation through a device placed inside the coronary sinus. In a significant number of individuals, in fact, the coronary sinus lies superior to the plane of the atrioventricular junction and the leaflet hinge line. In these cases, mitral annulus reduction through this percutaneous intervention may result in traction applied on the left atrial wall rather than on the hinge line of the posterior mitral leaflet, with relatively minor impact on annular area reduction and mitral regurgitation (Fig. 1.6).

The spatial arrangement between the hinge line, muscular crest of the left ventricle, coronary arteries, and coronary sinus is also important in surgical valve reconstruction, as the stitches used to sew the prosthetic ring must be placed on the atrial wall about 2 mm above the hinge line, in order to be attached to a more resilient tissue, securing the ring and simultaneously preserving the motion of the leaflet. In the new percutaneous direct annuloplasty strategies using a flexible ring (such as Cardioband [Valtech Cardio Ltd. for Edwards Lifesciences, Nyon, Switzerland]), the anchors must be placed into the muscular/fibrous tissue around the posterior annulus, 2–3 mm externally from the hinge line of the leaflet.

The absence of a continuous dense band of connective tissue makes the posterior annulus prone to dilatation. Moreover, it is also a frequent target of extensive calcifications, the so-called mitral annular calcification (MAC).

Fig. 1.5 (**a, b**) Two-dimensional (2D) transthoracic echocardiography (TTE) long-axis view showing the posterior leaflet insertion. In the magnified image of the structures inside the *red square* (**b**), the hinge line of the posterior leaflet is clearly seen. The *dotted red line* marks the atrioventricular groove, but the vessel running in the groove cannot be visualized because of insufficient spatial resolution. (**c, d**) 2D transesophageal echocardiography (TEE) images of the posterior leaflet insertion. Although TEE has better spatial resolution than TTE, vessels in the atrioventricular groove also cannot be distinguished. (**e, f**) 3D TEE of the mitral valve from an overhead perspective in early diastole (**e**) and end systole (**f**), showing how the posterior annulus (*arrows*) contributes to the reduction of annular area (sphincteric action) following the left ventricular contraction. *CS* coronary sinus

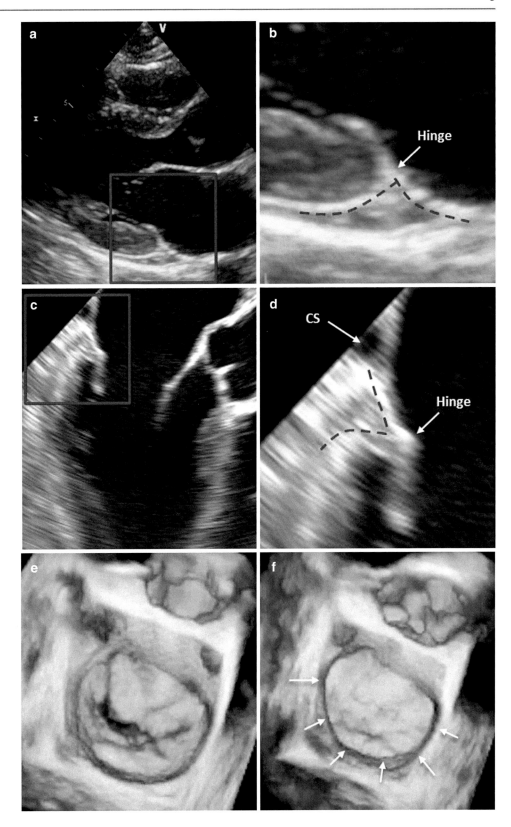

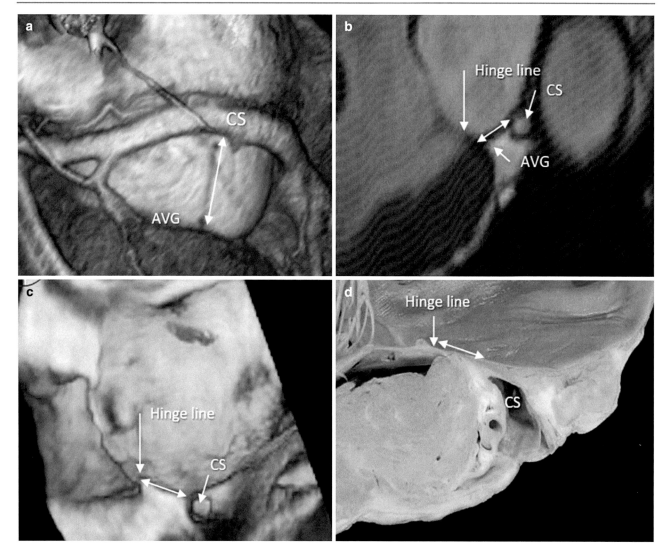

Fig. 1.6 The coronary sinus (CS) lies superior to the atrioventricular groove (AVG) and leaflet hinge line (*double-headed arrow*), as seen on CT volume-rendered acquisition (**a**), CMR SSFP sequence (**b**), 3D TEE (**c**), and an anatomic specimen (**d**)

Although often described as a passive, degenerative age-related process, accumulating evidence suggests that MAC is closely associated with vascular atherosclerosis and cardiovascular risk factors. MAC is also frequently observed in patients with renal failure, owing to abnormal calcium-phosphorus metabolism.

The Anterior Annulus

The anterior mitral annulus, considered as a band of connective tissue that anchors the anterior leaflet, simply ***does not exist***. From a ventricular perspective, the anterior leaflet is, in fact, in continuity with a sheet of fibrous tissue (called the *mitral-aortic curtain*, *mitral aortic continuity*, or *mitral aortic intervalvular fibrosa*), which continues imperceptibly into the left inter leaflet triangle. We will hereinafter refer to this area as the *mitral-aortic curtain*.

The mitral-aortic curtain is more or less rectangular and is delimited medially and laterally by two fibrous nodules, the right and left fibrous trigones. Compared with the body of the anterior mitral leaflet, this region presents a slight increase in thickness.

Seen from the atrial perspective, the mitral-aortic curtain comprises the atrial wall that extends up to the hinge line of the anterior mitral leaflet, which lies lower than the hinge line of the aortic leaflet. Thus, the space between the two hinge lines is occupied on the ventricular side by the mitral-aortic curtain (Fig. 1.7).

This region is well known to surgeons and imagers because in patients with aortic endocarditis or an aortic prosthesis, this area is predisposed to the development of abscess,

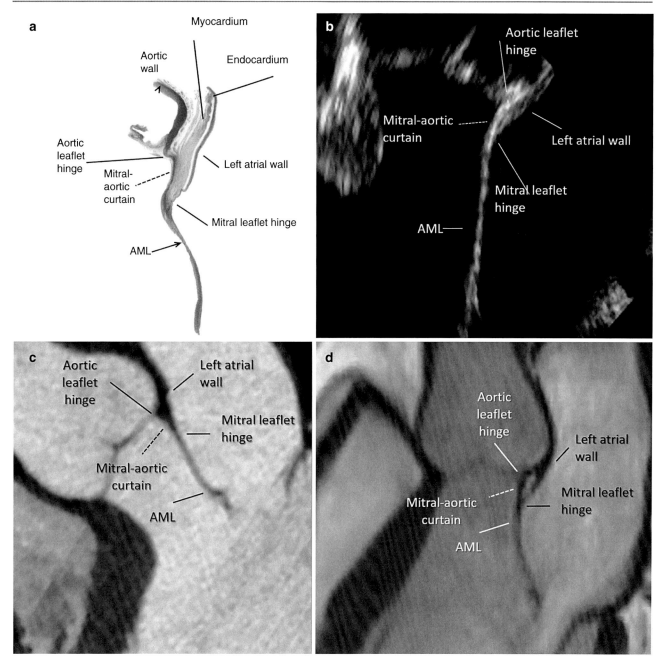

Fig. 1.7 (a) Histologic section of mitral-aortic curtain stained with elastic van Gieson stain showing fibrous tissue in red, myocardium in yellow, and elastic tissue in dark purple. (b) The corresponding echocardiographic image. The mitral aortic curtain is present only on the ventricular side of the anterior leaflet. On the atrial side, this space is occupied by atrial wall. (c) CT multiplanar images. Despite the high resolution power CT does not allow a clear distinction between aortic and atrial wall. (d) Unlike CT, CMR is capable of visualizing even a thin leaf of epicardial adipose tissue in between the two walls. *AML* anterior mitral leaflet

aneurysm, and perforation into the left atrium or the base of the anterior leaflet. The reason why the mitral-aortic curtain is a frequent target of aortic endocarditis is its continuity with the aortic leaflets. The infection may, in fact, propagate either by direct extension of the infected tissue inferiorly or as the result of infected regurgitant jet striking this region. Moreover, the mitral-aortic curtain is avascular, so it offers little resistance to infections. Exquisite images of this area can be obtained using 3D TEE from a ventricular perspective (Figs. 1.8 and 1.9).

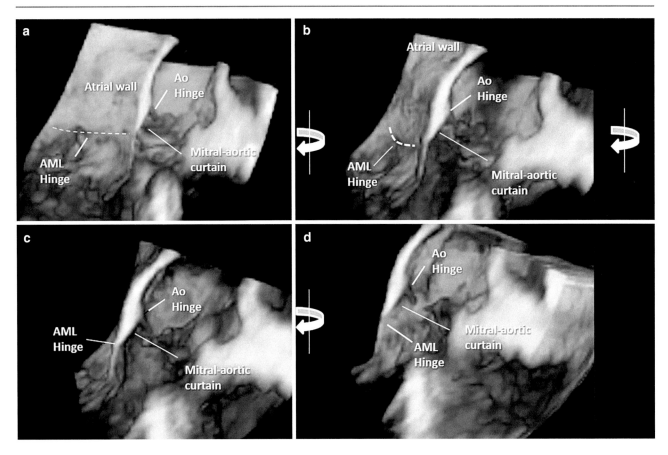

Fig. 1.8 The mitral-aortic curtain and its anatomical relationship with the anterior mitral leaflet (AML) hinge, the aortic (Ao) hinge, and the atrial wall, as illustrated by 3D TEE. (**a**) 3D zoom modality image showing the atrial aspect of mitral-aortic curtain from an oblique perspective. (**b–d**) Rotation right to left around Y-axis (*curve arrows*) progressively displays the mitral-aortic curtain from ventricular perspective

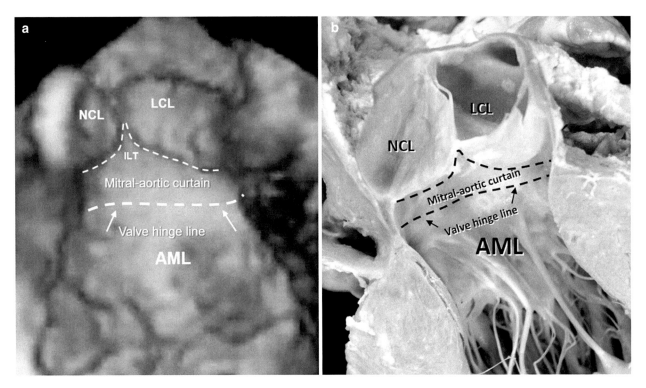

Fig. 1.9 (**a**) 3D TEE image from the ventricular perspective showing the anterior mitral leaflet (AML) in systole. The hinge line (*i.e.*, the fulcrum around which the leaflets move) is marked by the thicker dotted line, and the insertion of the aortic leaflets is marked by the thinner dotted line. The interleaflet triangle (ILT) is well recognizable between the aortic leaflets. (**b**) Anatomic specimen in similar display. *LCL* left coronary leaflet, *NCL* noncoronary leaflet

The Shape of the Annulus

In systole, the hinge of the mitral leaflets along the atrio-ventricular junction takes the form of a "D" (Fig. 1.10). The anteroposterior (or septal-lateral) diameter of the orifice is significantly shorter than the commissural diameter. In diastole, the annulus becomes more circular and the two diameters are almost equivalent. 3D TEE, being able to visu-alize the mitral complex from an overhead perspective, is certainly the best imaging technique to illustrate the shape of the annulus. What 3D TEE shows from this perspective is the hinge line of leaflets. This perspective is the same as the exposed view seen during cardiac surgery, so it takes the name of *surgical view*.

The three-dimensional saddle-shaped configuration of the annulus was described by Robert Levine and colleagues in

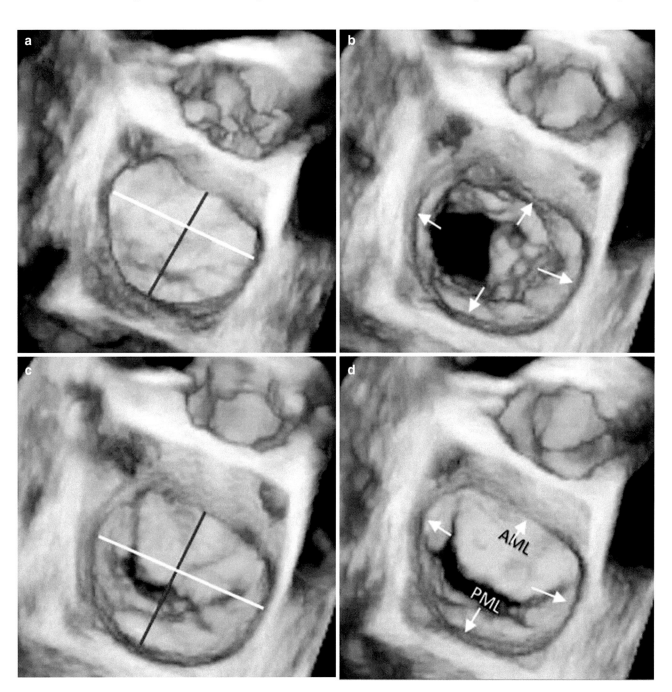

Fig. 1.10 The shape of the annulus as seen with 3D TEE at different time points of the cardiac cycle. (a) In mid-systole, the shape assumes an elliptical configuration (like a letter "D" lying down). The anteroposterior diameter (*red line*) is shorter than the commissural diameter (*white line*). (c) In late diastole, the annulus is almost circular. Thus, the anterior-posterior and the commissural diameters are equivalent. (b) and (d) are intermediate phases. *AML* anterior mitral leaflet, *PML* posterior mitral leaflet

the 1980s. Instead of a planar configuration, they reported variable heights of the hinge of the leaflets in relation to the apex, with the highest edge being located at the level of the midpoints of the anterior and posterior leaflets and the lowest edge at the commissural level. This description generated a profound conceptual reconsideration of the echocardiographic diagnosis of mitral valve prolapse. This configuration explains the reduced stress on the leaflets, and most of the rings currently used by surgeons are designed to respect this three-dimensional geometry. The best way to visualize the saddle-shaped aspect of the annulus is by using 2D slices obtained from the 3D data set. The hinge line is manually traced in several adjacent long-axis planes, and the reconstructed annulus is then displayed as a color-coded 3D-rendered surface (Fig. 1.11). It must be emphasized that both in the original paper and in current 3D TEE color-coded rendered surface reconstruction, the contour traced to reconstruct the saddle-shaped configuration is the hinge line of leaflets, rather than the annulus. Thus, the correct definition should refer to the *saddle-shaped configuration of the mitral hinge line*.

Annulus Motion

During the cardiac cycle, the mitral annulus (or more precisely, the leaflet hinge line) undergoes three types of motions: a sphincteric-like contraction, a translation motion, and an annular folding.

A *sphincteric-like contraction* occurs specifically at the level of the posterior annulus as a consequence of the contraction of basal helical fibers. The "sphincter" mechanism reduces the orifice area by 20–30%, thereby increasing the coaptation surface of the leaflets and ensuring perfect valve competence. The orifice area is minimum in mid to end systole (*see* Fig. 1.10a) and maximum in isovolumetric relaxation to early diastole (*see* Fig. 1.10c).

The *translation motion* is a consequence of the long-axis reduction of the left ventricle (LV); it is functionally linked to atrial and ventricular filling and emptying. In diastole, the annulus is pulled away from the LV apex, promoting LV filling by displacing a column of blood initially present in the left atrium beneath mitral leaflets. In systole, because the LV apex is fixed to the diaphragm by the pericardial sac,

Fig. 1.11 3D TEE color-coded rendered surface reconstruction of the saddle-shaped configuration of the annulus. (**a**) The operator follows the hinge line (*arrows*). The fulcrum (around which the leaflets open and close) is clearly visible (*arrows*). (**b–d**) Color-coded 3D rendered surface shows the saddle-shaped configuration from three different perspectives. Because the contour traced to reconstruct the saddle-shaped configuration is the hinge line of the leaflets, a better description should be the *saddle-shaped configuration of the mitral hinge line*. *A* anterior, *AL* anterior-lateral, *Ao* aorta, *P* posterior, *PM* posterior-medial

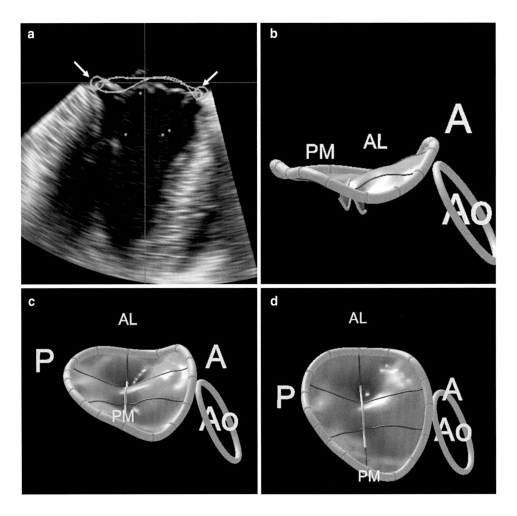

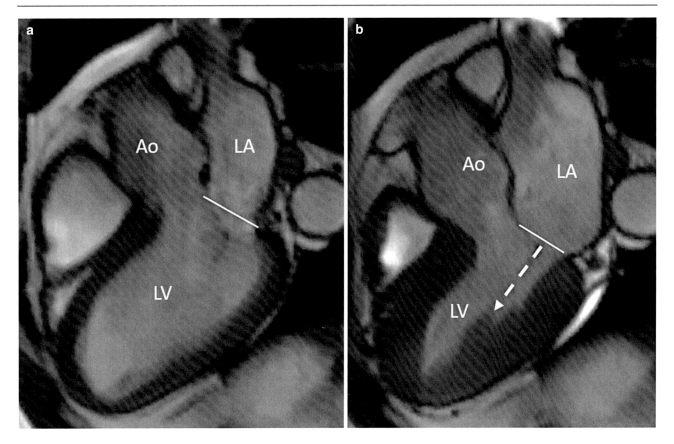

Fig. 1.12 (**a**, **b**) Frames captured from cine sequences of CMR, showing the movement of the mitral annulus towards the apex

the longitudinal LV shortening causes the base of the heart (and consequently of the annulus) to move towards the apex. This longitudinal shortening of the left ventricle reflects the contribution of the contraction of endocardial and epicardial muscular fibers, which have a prevalent longitudinal/oblique orientation. This motion displaces a column of blood, which is ejected into the aorta and simultaneously enlarges the left atrium, causing a drop in atrial pressure that facilitates the pulmonary venous return. This apical excursion of 5–10 mm has been shown to generate at least one fourth of the LV stroke volume. The excursion of the annulus can be best appreciated (and measured) in cine CMR sequences using a long-axis view plane (Fig. 1.12). It must be said that the degree of displacement of the anterior and posterior portions of the leaflet hinge line is not equal; the anterior annulus is tethered by the aortic root and translates less than the posterior annulus.

The *annular folding*, an accentuation of the saddle-shaped configuration, occurs during the systole. This conformational change avoids leaflet distortion along the hinge line, a potential consequence of annular contraction. As mentioned above, an accentuated saddle-shaped configura-tion blunts the stress on leaflets that occurs as LV pressure rises. Another mechanism that favors the annular folding is the expansion of the aortic root, which displaces the mitral-aortic curtain posteriorly.

Mitral Leaflets

The most remarkable components of the mitral valve are undoubtedly the leaflets. The well-known description of the mitral valve with two leaflets is actually imprecise from a strict anatomical point of view. The two incisures, called *commissures* (a name that literally refers to the junction line between two adjacent structures), which divide the valve tissue into two halves, *do not* reach the hinge line. Thus, the presence of valve tissue along the entire circumference of the hinge creates an anatomical continuity between the two leaflets, thus making the mitral valve a continuous, uninterrupted veil. Because these incisures are consistently present in any normal mitral valve, however, the term *bicuspid valve* is justified. Therefore, we continue to describe the mitral valve as having two leaflets and two commissures.

The Commissures

The commissures are the deepest incisures of the valve leaflets. Because of the oblique orientation of the longitudinal axis of the left ventricle inside the thorax (from right to left, from top to bottom, and from posterior to anterior), the anterior-lateral commissure is higher than the posterior-medial commissure. The position of the commissures can be easily appreciated by using a new technology based on the "fusion" of fluoroscopy and 3D TEE (Fig. 1.13).

The unique chordal arrangement arising from the tip of the papillary muscles as a single stem, branching radially and embracing the commissures, is used by anatomists to define the limits of the commissural area. Frequently, the commissural tissue takes the shape of a small Y-shaped segment called a *commissural scallop*. In the same mitral valve, one commissure may have a small commissural scallop while the other is represented by a simple strip of valve tissue. Whatever the configuration, this additional tissue is critical for obtaining a sufficient area of coaptation in this region. The best way to visualize the commissures remains 3D TEE, in which both commissures are clearly depicted from an overhead perspective (Fig. 1.14).

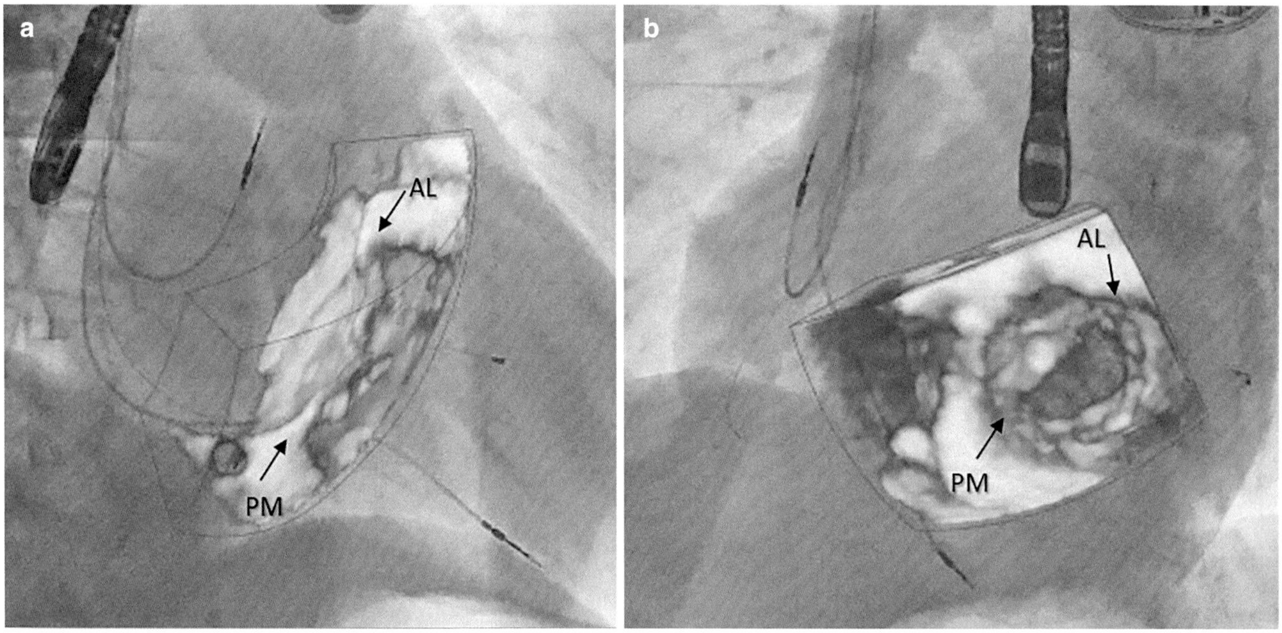

Fig. 1.13 Fusion images of fluoroscopy and 3D TEE showing the positions of the anterior-lateral commissure (AL) and posterior-medial commissure (PM) of the mitral valve, in a right anterior oblique projection (**a**) and in a left anterior oblique projection (**b**)

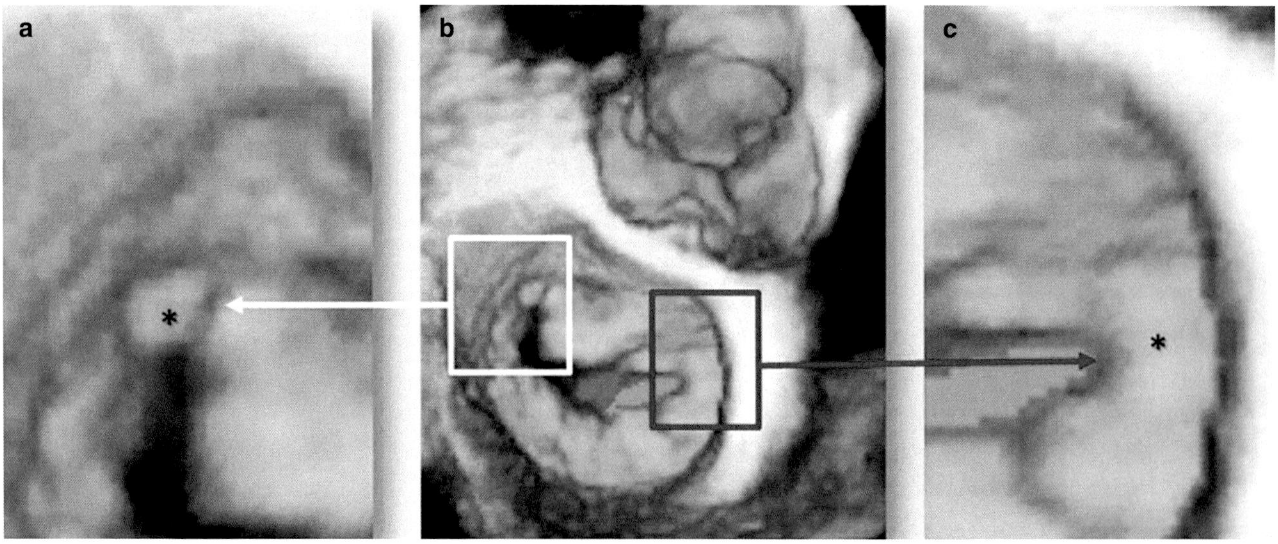

Fig. 1.14 (**a**) Magnified 3D TEE image (white square from panel **b**) showing the Y-shaped anterior-lateral commissure (*asterisk*). (**c**) Magnified image (red square from panel **b**) showing the posterior-medial commissure without any well-defined commissural scallop (*asterisk*)

The Leaflets

The commissures divide the mitral valve into two leaflets: *the anterior leaflet* (or, given its strict continuity with the aortic valve, the *aortic leaflet*) and the *posterior leaflet* (or, given its strict continuity with the margin of the left ventricle, the *mural leaflet*). The anterior leaflet has almost a triangular shape, and its hinge line occupies approximately one third of the annulus. The length from the hinge point to the free margin varies from 1.5 to 2.5 cm. The free margin is usually devoid of incisures (Fig. 1.15a). The posterior leaflet reveals a relatively quadrangular shape, and its

hinge line occupies the remaining two thirds of the mitral annulus (Fig. 1.15b). The distance between the insertion and the free margin is shorter than for the anterior leaflet, measuring less than 1 cm, but given its longer hinge line, the areas of the two leaflets are almost equal. In contrast to the anterior leaflet, the posterior leaflet usually has two indentations, which divide the leaflet into three parts called *scallops*. According to Carpentier's classification, these scallops, from lateral to medial, are named P1, P2, and P3. These indentations usually extend as deep as half of the distance between the free margin and the hinge line of the posterior leaflet and are supported by numerous chordae. The scallops have a

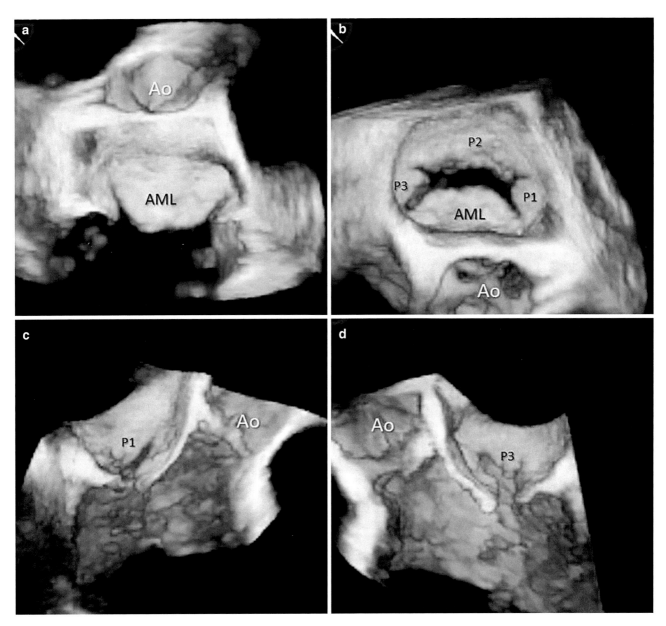

Fig. 1.15 (**a–d**) 3D TEE images of mitral leaflets as visualized from different perspectives (**a**, cropped image of surgical perspective; **b**, anterior perspective from overhead; **c** and **d**, cropped image of long-axis perspective showing P1 and P3 scallop). P1, P2, and P3 denote the three scallops of the posterior mitral leaflet. *AML* anterior mitral leaflet, *Ao* aorta

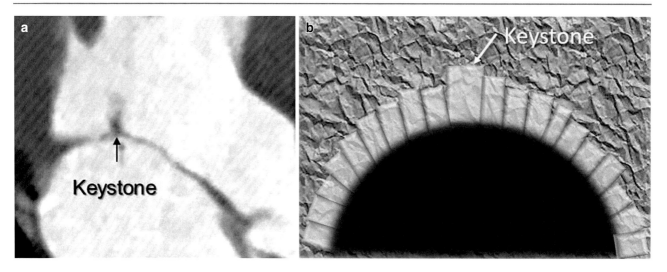

Fig. 1.16 (**a**, **b**) The keystone mechanism of leaflet coaptation attenuates the stress on the leaflets and chordal apparatus

semi-elliptical shape, and frequently, the central one is the largest. They act exactly as the commissures, facilitating a larger opening in diastole and favoring an effective closure in systole. Other smaller incisures may subdivide a single scallop into subunits. The term *cleft* should be used to indicate a deeper indentation that extends from the free edge to the hinge line and, when present, results in regurgitation. Clefts are usually present in degenerative valve disease (large prolapse or Barlow disease). The best imaging technique to explore the leaflets is the 3D TEE, in which the valve can be visualized in its entirety.

The ventricular surface of the two leaflets can be divided into two portions: the rough zone (pars rugosa) and the clear, translucent zone (pars liscia). The rough zone is thicker and has an irregular surface owing to the insertion of chordae tendineae onto the underside of the leaflets. This area is wider in the central zone of both leaflets and gradually fades as it approaches the commissures. In the anterior leaflet, the clear zone is rather thin, translucent, relatively wide, and elastic. In systole, it may therefore acquire a convex shape towards the atrial cavity. This systolic shape, though frequently misdiagnosed as a prolapse, is far from being pathological. Instead, it is rather beneficial, because the convexity reduces the mechanical stress by distributing the systolic pressure more evenly. In the posterior leaflet, the clear zone is a narrow, flexible band. Characteristically, the rough zone corresponds, on its atrial surface, to the coaptation surface of the valve leaflets. The coaptation surface is critical for a perfect valve competence. The leaflets "coapt" over a height of 6–8 mm, thus endowing the valve with a kind of "valvular reserve" that preserves valve function even in the event of "moderate" annular dilatation. The coaptation forms an arc-shaped closure line, which is obliquely situated relative to the orthogonal plane of the body. The posterior leaflet provides an anchor against which the anterior leaflet abuts

to maintain valve competence. This "keystone" mechanism (as for an ancient arch made of stones) considerably reduces the tension and the pressure on the leaflets and the chordal apparatus, as the LV pressure is exerted simultaneously on the two opposite sides of the leaflets (Fig. 1.16). Because of the different lengths of the anterior and posterior leaflets, in normal individuals, this area is asymmetrical, with an anterior leaflet dominance. Echocardiography, CMR, and CT scans may offer excellent images of the coaptation surface (Fig. 1.17).

Microstructure of the Leaflets

The leaflets are tacitly perceived as two flaps of inert tissue, but this belief is far from accurate. The mitral valve leaflets in an adult must open and close over 100,000 times a day (more than three trillion times in a lifetime) in order to maintain unidirectional blood flow. This goal could not be achieved with inert tissue. Mitral leaflets are made of living tissue with a highly organized connective tissue system that provides unique mechanical properties. Indeed, cross sections reveal three well-defined layers: the atrial is on the flow side of the leaflet, the spongiosa in the middle, and the fibrosa or ventricularis on the ventricular side. This three-layered structure is covered on both the ventricular and the atrial surfaces with a single layer of endothelial cells. Each layer has different molecular characteristics, which impart unique mechanical properties to the leaflets. The *atrialis,* for example, contains lamellar collagen and elastin sheets, thus forming a robust yet elastic network that counteracts the systolic deformation in systole and enables elastic recoil in diastole. The *spongiosa* contains loose connective fibers and glycosaminoglycans, which counteract the compressive forces generated by coaptation by absorbing tension and

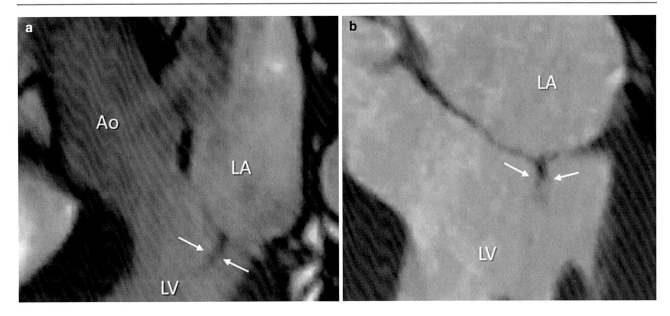

Fig. 1.17 CMR image (**a**) and CT scan (**b**) showing the coaptation surface (*arrows*) in systole. *Ao* aorta, *LA* left atrium, *LV* left ventricle

friction between the layers, like a lubricant cushion. Finally, the *fibrosa*, made of collagen densely packed in robust fibers and arranged parallel to the free margin of the leaflet, confers strength and stiffness. At sites of chordal insertion, the fibrosa is in continuity with a robust cylindrical strand of collagen fibers that form the "core" of the chordae tendineae. This architecture faces the high LV pressure with a gradual transition of forces between leaflets and chordae (Fig. 1.18).

The most striking feature of the microstructure of the mitral leaflets is the cellular population. Mitral leaflets contain mainly two types of cells: valvular endothelial cells, covering the leaflet surface, and the interstitial cells, with at least five different types distributed throughout the leaflets. Both cellular components are essential to maintain the matrix network that forms the mechanical scaffold to sustain the dynamic activity of the leaflets and to confer robustness and durability.

Notably, in medical textbooks and guidelines, functional mitral regurgitation (both ischemic and non-ischemic) is described as a "secondary" regurgitation. This term emphasizes the fact that mitral regurgitation is a result of geometric distortion of the papillary muscles due to the enlargement of the left ventricle, while the valve leaflets and chordal apparatus are structurally normal. Consequently, therapies have focused on reducing annular and ventricular remodeling. But this paradigm is not completely true. Indeed, preclinical and clinical studies have shown leaflets that are larger and thicker than normal in patients with longstanding functional mitral regurgitation. In other words, the leaflets are not innocent bystanders in functional mitral regurgitation. Mechanical stretching of the leaflets may activate fibroblast-like cell populations, which increase collagen production and render the

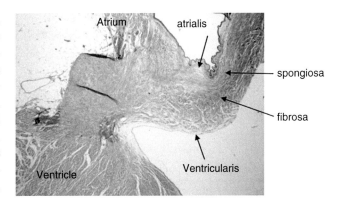

Fig. 1.18 Histologic section through mitral leaflet (elastic van Gieson stain)

leaflets larger and thicker in order to compensate for annular dilation and/or geometric remodeling of the left ventricle. The knowledge of this "adaptive" mechanism (though still at an early stage) shifts away from the well-accepted model in which the leaflets are structurally normal and the insufficiency is a matter of unbalanced closing against tethering forces due to abnormal LV geometry. The new paradigm focuses on leaflet remodeling. The histological remodeling of leaflets leading to active valve enlargement can be seen as an adaptive mechanism to restore effective coaptation, but it is not illogical to consider the possibility that excessive remodeling may result in a stiffer leaflet with decreased mobility, which in turn may interfere with effective closure and exacerbate mitral regurgitation. Thus the mechanisms of functional mitral regurgitation are likely to be more complex than previously thought. Indeed, it seems to be not simply a balance between closing versus tethering forces but also an adaptive versus a maladaptive fibrosis. As effective closure requires thin, flexible, and elastic leaflets that expand nearly 15% in systole to form a coaptational seal, stiffer leaflets may increase mitral regurgitation, rather than reducing it.

Chordae Tendineae

The simplest and most effective classification divides the chordae into three categories: the first-order or *marginal* chordae, the second-order *strut or stay* chordae, and the third-order *basal* chordae (Fig. 1.19). Despite marked variability in number and distribution among individuals, the general design of the chordal apparatus is rather constant. The chordae originate from the tip or heads of the papillary muscles, as single stems that split radially into several branches. Only the basal chordae may originate directly from the left ventricular wall. Before inserting into the leaflets, the chordal branches form numerous interconnections, thus ensuring a balanced distribution of forces and robust structural stability.

These three types of chordae exert different functions. *The marginal chordae* insert on the free margin of the leaflets, and the rupture of a main marginal chorda is responsible for flail and severe mitral regurgitation. Commissural chordae are considered to be part of marginal chordae. The *strut* or *stay chordae* are attached close to the boundary between the rough and the clear zone on both leaflets. Of particular interest are two strut chordae that are inserted on the anterior leaflet at an angle of 45°. They are located at a distance approximately one third of the way from the free edge and two thirds from the annulus; sometimes they divide

before their insertion into two or three branches. These chordae are particularly thick and robust. Indeed, in the animal model, the tension exerted during systole on these chordae is three times higher than the force exerted on the marginal chordae, and these chordae remain tense during the entire cardiac cycle. The function of these chordae is still not completely understood. Their main function does not seem to be the prevention of mitral regurgitation. In the animal model, transection of these chordae does not result in either mitral regurgitation or changes in leaflet coaptation; it results in global LV systolic dysfunction. In fact, these chordae maintain a fibrous connection between the mitral valve and the papillary muscles and may contribute to the preservation of LV geometry by favoring long-axis LV shortening. They also reduce the motion of the peripheral part of the anterior mitral leaflet, thus leaving the central part more mobile. In systole, therefore, the leaflet takes a concave shape on the side of the LV outflow tract, which facilitates the blood flow transit towards the aorta. In diastole, the concavity faces the inflow tract and facilitates the inflow of the blood into the left ventricle.

It is interesting to note that in the setting of secondary mitral regurgitation of ischemic or idiopathic origin, strut chordae are believed to exacerbate leaflet tethering. Therefore, some authors have suggested the transection of strut chordae as an adjunct technique to valve annuloplasty to improve leaflet coaptation. This mechanism has decreased mitral regurgitation in the experimental setting, but surgeons remain skeptical about implementing the procedure in standard mitral surgery because of their awareness that the cutting of the anterior strut chordae may have detrimental effects on LV function.

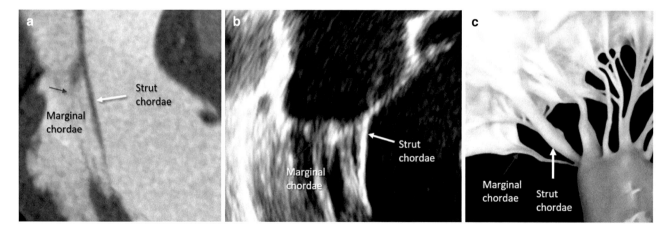

Fig. 1.19 CT scan (**a**), echocardiogram (**b**), and anatomic specimen (**c**) showing the strut chordae (*white arrow*) and the marginal chordae (*red arrow*)

The basal chordae originate directly from the ventricular wall and insert only on the posterior leaflet. Theoretically, the function of the basal chordae is to reduce the mobility of the leaflet by anchoring the valve to the ventricular wall. The absence of similar chordae on the anterior leaflet is due to the fact that the basal portion of the anterior leaflet continues with the mitral aortic curtain and has no anatomical connection with the ventricular wall.

Microstructure of Chordae Tendineae

The chordae tendineae consist of a core of densely packed collagen fibers in continuity with the fibrosa of the leaflets, surrounded by a layer of loose connective tissue of elastic fibers interspersed with collagen fibrils, and an outer layer of endothelial cells. This histological composition allows sustaining of the cyclic stress to which the chordae are continuously subjected. Moreover, the presence of vessels in the middle layer of the thicker chordae, running longitudinally from the papillary muscles to the mitral leaflets, strongly indicate that chordae tendineae are not simply passive collagenous structures, but represent live tissue with its own metabolism and an additional important role in leaflet nutrition. Moreover, in functional mitral regurgitation, chordal elongation may occur as part of the adaptive process to preserve leaflet coaptation.

Papillary Muscles

The papillary muscles (PM) originate from the apical third of the left ventricle and are usually organized into the anterior-lateral and the posterior-medial groups, which are positioned just below the corresponding commissures. Each of the two groups of PMs gives rise to a dozen or so main chordae tendineae, which insert into the medial and lateral halves of the anterior and posterior leaflets respectively. Considerable differences in shape and size have been described among individuals. Papillary muscles have been described as arising from the inner part of the left ventricle wall as a single body or as two or three bodies. The axis of these bodies is usually parallel to the long axis of the left ventricular cavity. Generally, the thickness of the PM matches with the thickness of the LV free wall, with a slight difference between the two PM (the anterior-lateral PM being larger than the posterior-medial PM), but considerable variation in size,

length, and configuration (single PM with or without multiple heads or multiple PMs) may occur.

In the 1960s, PM came to be appreciated as an essential component of the mitral valve apparatus, with a role in the closure process of the mitral leaflets. When the LV contracts and shortens, the PM contract and shorten as well, keeping the distance between the tips of the PM and the leaflets constant. The contraction of the PM prevents eversion of the leaflets during systole. The best imaging modalities to appreciate PM shortening are undoubtedly CMR and echocardiography.

Transient isolated PM ischemia or necrosis and fibrosis may result in leaflet prolapse with mitral regurgitation. In such a case, the regurgitation (and murmur) starts after the isometric contraction, when the ventricle begins to shorten. Involvement of both the PM and surrounding LV wall in the ischemic process causes asymmetric tethering of the leaflet. In these cases, the consequent mitral regurgitation (and murmur) starts at the beginning of the isometric contraction.

It is important to discuss PM vascularization, which may be responsible for different clinical presentations. Indeed, myocardial infarction involving the posterior myocardial wall usually results in necrosis of the posterior-medial PM, while anterior myocardial infarction may spare the anterior-lateral PM. In fact, the anterior-lateral PM has a dual blood supply from both the anterior descending and the circumflex coronary arteries, whereas the posterior-medial PM is dependent only on the coronary artery that gives origin to the posterior descending coronary artery. Because of this "asymmetric" blood supply, the postero-medial PM is considered to be more vulnerable to an ischemic insult.

Several articles and textbooks have described PM as arising directly from the compact myocardium, but this belief was recently challenged by CT scans and 2D echocardiography revealing that PM arise from a network of trabeculations rather than from a single pillar originating from the compact myocardium layer (Fig. 1.20). Such an arrangement of the PM suggests that by distributing the systolic pressure more uniformly on a larger base, a broad, mesh-like architecture with multiple points of attachment could protect PM from ventricular pressure more effectively than a pillar-like attachment. Furthermore, multiple trabecular origins allow PM to draw blood supply from numerous pathways, thus ensuring diffuse collateral perfusion protecting against ischemic insults.

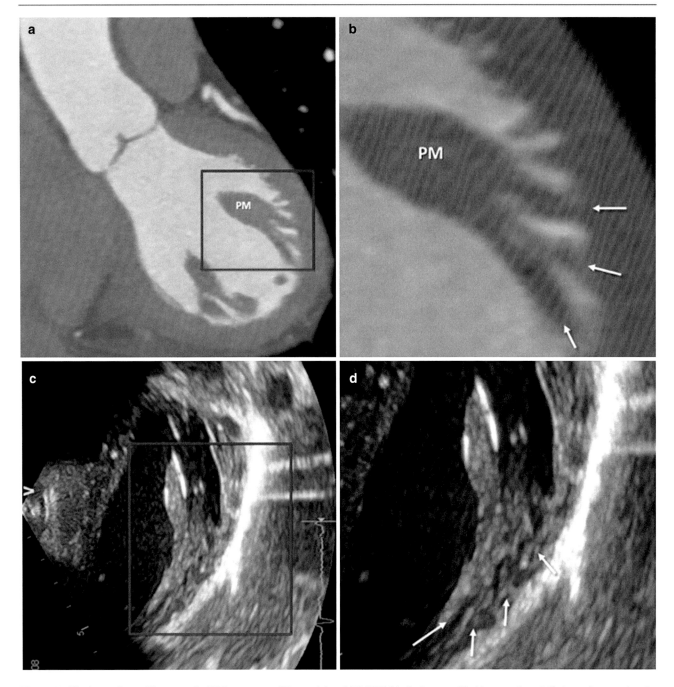

Fig. 1.20 The base of a papillary muscle (PM), seen on a CT scan (**a**) and 2D TTE (**c**). In the magnified images (**b** and **d**), it can be seen that the PM arises from a network of trabeculations (*arrows*), not as a single pillar from the compact myocardium

Suggested Reading

Angelini A, Ho SY, Anderson RH, Davies MJ, Becker AE. A histological study of the atrioventricular junction in hearts with normal and prolapsed leaflets of the mitral valve. Br Heart J. 1988;59:712–6.

Becker AE, de Wit APM. The mitral valve apparatus: a spectrum of normality relevant to mitral valve prolapse. Br Heart J. 1980;42:680–9.

Carpentier A, Deloche A, Dauptain J, Soyer R, Blondeau P, Piwnica A, et al. A new reconstructive operation for correction of mitral and tricuspid insufficiency. J Thorac Cardiovasc Surg. 1971;61:1–13.

Ho SY. Anatomy of the mitral valve. Heart. 2002;88(Suppl 4):iv5–10.

Levine RA, Handschumacher MD, Sanfilippo AJ, Hagege AA, Harrigan O, Marshall JE, et al. Three-dimensional echocardiographic reconstruction of the mitral valve, with implications for the diagnosis of mitral valve prolapse. Circulation. 1989;80:589–98.

Perloff JK, Roberts WC. The mitral valve apparatus. Functional anatomy of mitral regurgitation. Circulation. 1972;46:227–39.

Ranganathan N, Lam JHC, Wigle ED, Silver MD. Morphology of the human mitral valve. II. The valve leaflets. Circulation. 1970;41:459–67.

Victor S, Nayak VM. Definition and function of commissures, slits and scallops of the mitral valve: analysis in 100 hearts. Asia Pacific J Thorac Cardiovasc Surg. 1994;3:10–6.

Yacoub M. Anatomy of the mitral valve, chordae and cusps. In: Kalmanson D, editor. The mitral valve. London: Edward Arnold; 1976. p. 15–20.

The Aortic Root

Francesco F. Faletra, Enrico Ferrari, Giovanni Pedrazzini,
Siew Yen Ho, and Jagat Narula

The term *aortic root* (or *arterial root*) refers to the entirety of the aortic valve from its position at the left ventricular outlet to its junction with the tubular portion of the ascending aorta. Thus, the functioning valve is much more complex than only leaflets or flaps passively guarding the ventricular exit. The first "scientific" report of the sophisticated architecture of the aortic root dates back to the writings and drawings of Leonardo da Vinci. He drew three small bulges at the base of the aorta and correctly theorized their function, picturing the "eddy currents" or vortexes between leaflets and sinuses. Two hundred years later, these three bulges would be given the name "Valsalva's sinuses" by Antonio Maria Valsalva, an Italian anatomist. In reality, Valsalva was more interested in the anatomy of the hearing system, and his famous book, *De Aure Humana Tractatus* ("The Book of the Human Ear"), remained the gold standard on the subject for more than a century. He had also discovered an original method of pressurizing the middle ear, the Valsalva maneuver, which is still widely used. Valsalva performed many dissections of the chest, and described the sinuses of Valsalva as "pouches of the aorta and the pulmonary artery opposite the flaps of the

semilunar valves." He was intrigued by the uniform presence of sinuses in a variety of birds and mammalians and concluded that the sinuses must have a common important function in these living species.

Despite this longstanding interest, until a few decades ago the aortic root was considered only an inert, unidirectional conduit between the left ventricle and the ascending aorta. Moreover, because aortic leaflets do not have an extensive attachment with the ventricular myocardium, their function was thought to be entirely passive, driven by pressure fluctuations between the left ventricle and the ascending aorta. Whenever the pressure generated by ventricular contraction exceeded the pressure in the ascending aorta, the leaflets would open, allowing for unidirectional blood flow, and similarly, whenever the ventricular pressure decreased below aortic pressure, the leaflets would close, preventing backflow. Cardiologists may have disregarded the anatomy of the aortic root because of this apparent structural and functional simplicity.

The advent of aortic valve-sparing surgery, first performed by Tyron David in 1992, and transcatheter aortic valve implantation (TAVI), first performed in humans by Alain Cribier in 2002, renewed the interest of the cardiology community in the anatomy of the aortic root. Both procedures require a systematic and thorough analysis of the fine anatomy of the valve apparatus and its components; the aortic root was no longer considered a simple, passive conduit, but rather a sophisticated ensemble of various anatomical entities strategically placed to act as a whole.

A detailed examination of the aortic root architecture reveals how this valvular apparatus is extremely complex and effective. The shape of the root, which is similar to the truncal conus, and the cyclic adaptation of both the ventriculo-arterial junction and the sinutubular junction function to maintain laminar flow of large, intermittent blood volumes. The distensibility of the aortic wall, the pliability of the leaflets, and their coronet-shaped insertion accommodate large blood flow variations (up to five times) without

F. F. Faletra (✉)
Non-invasive Cardiovascular Imaging Department, Fondazione Cardiocentro Ticino, Lugano, Switzerland
e-mail: Francesco.Faletra@cardiocentro.org

E. Ferrari
Cardiac Surgery Department, Fondazione Cardiocentro Ticino, Lugano, Switzerland
e-mail: enrico.ferrari@cardiocentro.org

G. Pedrazzini
Cardiology Department, Fondazione Cardiocentro Ticino, Lugano, Switzerland
e-mail: giovanni.pedrazzini@cardiocentro.org

S. Y. Ho
Royal Brompton Hospital, Sydney Street, London, UK
e-mail: yen.ho@imperial.ac.uk

J. Narula
Icahn School of Medicine at Mount Sinai, New York, NY, USA
e-mail: narula@mountsinai.org

© Springer Nature Switzerland AG 2020
F. F. Faletra et al. (eds.), *Atlas of Non-Invasive Imaging in Cardiac Anatomy*, https://doi.org/10.1007/978-3-030-35506-7_2

significant increase in the ventriculo-arterial gradient. Moreover, the shape of the aortic sinuses, with a diastolic three-lobe configuration, creates a low-stress environment that guarantees life-long leaflet durability. For these functions, the aortic root deserves the title of the "fifth chamber" of the heart. This chapter describes the current understanding of functional aortic root anatomy, illustrated by echocardiography, CT scans, and cardiac magnetic resonance (CMR) imaging.

The "Babel" of Terminology

To fully appreciate the anatomy of the aortic root, a fundamental prerequisite is the adoption of a unified nomenclature. The moving parts of the aortic root are named *leaflets* or *cusps*, two different names for the same structure. The online version of the "Terminologia Anatomica" 1998 uses the term *cusp*. The anatomists who chose this term noticed a similarity between the aortic valve, viewed from a ventricular perspective and in closed position, and the surface of a molar tooth (called a *cusp*). The term *leaflet* has a meaning of "small leaf," a name that describes a thin, pliable layer and that perfectly fits the leaflet valve morphology. This chapter will use the term *leaflet* to describe the mobile parts of the aortic root (the valve), even though their composition may be referred to as *unicuspid*, *bicuspid*, or *tricuspid*.

The term *commissure* results from the Latin word *commissura*, indicating the point or the line where two structures, anatomical parts, or bodies join each other. Thus, the zone of leaflet apposition should be described as a *commissure*, but *commissure* may also indicate the angle between two lips or eyelids, and this second definition reflects the current use of the term. This chapter uses the term *commissure* to identify the most distal (superior) points of leaflet insertion on the aortic wall, but the remaining area, where leaflets meet, is called the *zone of apposition or coaptation*.

The term *aortic annulus* indicates the anatomical line where the aortic valve leaflets attach to the wall of the aortic root. The Latin word *anulus*, translated in English as *annulus*, means "ring," but a fibrous ring that holds leaflets on the aortic wall does not exist. This fact was again emphasized by McAlpine, who wrote in 1975 that the term *annulus* as applied to heart valves is "ill-founded—no such structures are to be found." Instead, the semilunar-shaped aortic leaflets are anchored to dense connective tissue that takes the shape of a crown. To describe the insertion of the valve leaflets in the aortic wall, we will therefore use the term *hinge line* instead of *annulus*. The circumference obtained by joining the lowest point of this hinge line (nadirs), although neither anatomically or histologically distinct, has surged to be of clinical relevance in the TAVI era. Measurements of this virtual basal plane allow for correct sizing of the valve. Because this region does not have any anatomical boundary, we agree with most recent literature, which defines this circumference as a "virtual annulus." On the other hand, standard prosthetic heart valves are traditionally sutured to a sort of "ring area" lying between the nadirs of the sinuses and midway to the commissures. This area defines the sizing position for a surgical valve prosthesis. Because surgeons suture prostheses in a circular manner, using the term "surgical annulus" to refer to this "ring area" does not seem to be illogical. Moreover, it provides a precise reference point when the prosthesis is sutured in a *supra-annular* position. This chapter uses the terms *crown-shaped hinge line*, *virtual annulus*, and *surgical annulus* with the above-mentioned meanings.

The terminology used in this chapter for the aortic sinuses—*left-coronary*, *right-coronary*, and *non-coronary*—is the most appropriate. Some may disagree because of the rare case of both main coronary arteries arising from the same sinus or, even more rarely, from the non-coronary sinus. Traditionally, anatomists have named the sinuses *anterior* (for right-coronary), *right posterior* (for non-coronary), and *left posterior* (for left-coronary). In normal hearts, the main right and left coronary arteries arise from the right-coronary and left-coronary sinuses respectively, and these are behind the pulmonary outflow tract, whereas the non-coronary sinus is well posterior. Some authors suggest the use of the terms *right*, *left*, and *non-facing* coronary sinuses, especially in congenitally malformed hearts where the aortic and pulmonary roots are in abnormal spatial relationships. Arterial relationships are normal in the vast majority of patients, however, so anomalous origin of the coronary arteries is seldom encountered, and this chapter uses the simple terminology of *left-coronary*, *right-coronary*, and *non-coronary*.

Terms such as *ventriculo-arterial junction*, *hemodynamic ventriculo-arterial junction*, or *anatomic/histological ventriculo-arterial junction*, used to describe the border between the ventricular myocardium and the fibroelastic structure of the aortic root, can appear ambiguous because they refer to a circle that includes not only muscular tissue but also two fibrous components, the mitral-aortic curtain and the membranous septum. These structures are discussed later.

Finally, the term *aortic valve* is used commonly to refer to the leaflets only, but rarely is applied to the entire aortic root. Although this latter "extensive" meaning of *aortic valve* incorporates the notion that other components contribute to the leaflets' function, we prefer the use of the term *aortic valve* to refer exclusively to the three leaflets. Therefore, when the aortic leaflets are surgically excised, the aortic valve "de facto" is no longer present.

The Position of the Aortic Root

When the base of the heart is viewed from an overhead perspective, the aortic root is the cardiac centerpiece, partially wedged between the orifices of the tricuspid and mitral valves (Fig. 2.1).

Viewed from an anteroposterior plane, the aortic root lies on the right, behind the right ventricular outflow tract and in front of the atria. The angle between the aortic root and the right ventricular outflow tract is approximately 60°, whereas the nadir of the valve sinuses lies in a plane that has an angle of 30° compared with the horizontal line (Fig. 2.2). Because of its central location in the heart, the aortic root is contiguous with all four cardiac chambers and valves.

The proximity of the non-coronary sinus to the interatrial septum (IAS) is well known to interventional cardiologists.

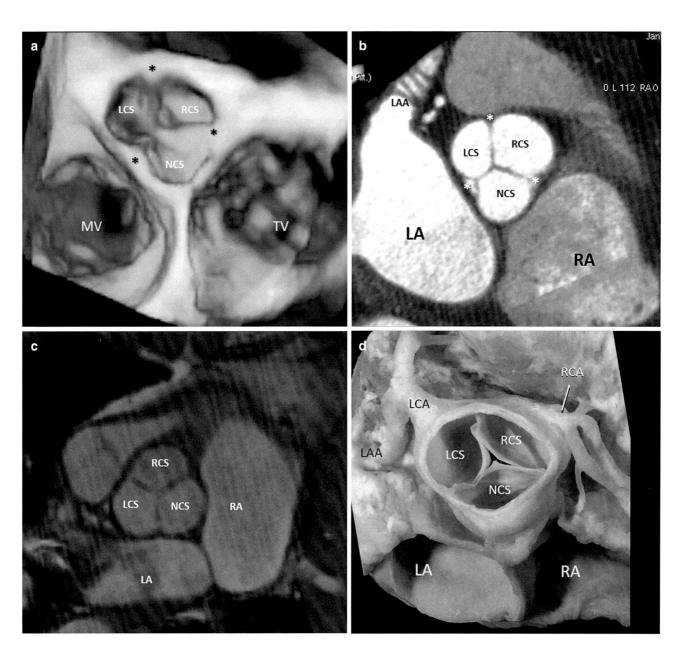

Fig. 2.1 The aortic root, wedged between the mitral valve (MV) and the tricuspid valve (TV), as shown in a three-dimensional transesophageal echocardiography (3D TEE) image from an overhead perspective (**a**) and a CT cross-section slice (**b**). The *asterisks* indicate the commissures. (**c**) Similar perspective in CMR. An anatomic specimen (**d**) also shows the origins of the left and right coronary arteries. *LA* left atrium, *LAA* left atrial appendage, *LCA* left coronary artery, *LCS* left-coronary sinus, *NCS* non-coronary sinus, *RA* right atrium, *RCA* right coronary artery, *RCS* right-coronary sinus

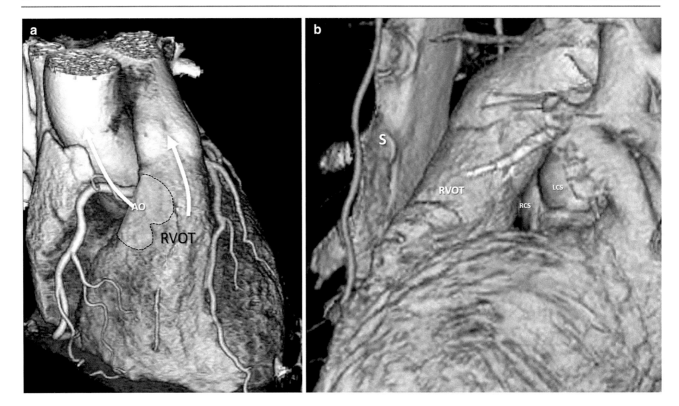

Fig. 2.2 (**a**) CT volume rendering image in anteroposterior projection, showing the position of the aortic root (AO) (delineated by the *black dotted line*) posterior to the right ventricular outflow tract (RVOT). The AO lies posteriorly and rightward of the RVOT. *Curved arrows* indicate the different directions of the aortic root and RVOT. (**b**) CT-assisted electronic cast in lateral projection; the right-coronary sinus (RCS) and the left-coronary sinus (LCS) face the RVOT. *S* sternum

When they puncture the IAS or close an atrial septal defect with a device, the risk of damaging the aortic wall is not negligible, especially if the aortic root is dilated. Moreover, because of its position, the left- and non-coronary sinuses may bulge into the left atrium, and the right- and non-coronary sinuses may bulge into the right atrium (Fig. 2.3).

The Components of the Aortic Root

The aortic root is composed of five key components:the ventriculo-arterial junction, the crescent-shaped hinge lines of semilunar leaflets, the sinuses, the leaflets, and the sinutubular junction.

The Ventriculo-Arterial Junction

The *anatomic* ventriculo-arterial junction is the point at which the left ventricular myocardium meets the fibroelastic wall of the aortic root. Unlike the right ventriculo-arterial junction, where the pulmonary leaflets are entirely supported by the muscular tissue of the subpulmonary infundibulum, the muscular component represents only 60% of the left ventriculo-arterial junction. The muscular myocardium rises up toward the commissure between the right-coronary sinus and left-coronary sinus. Because it extends above the nadir of the right and left leaflet hinge line, small segments of ventricular myocardium remain present in the right and left sinuses where the transition from the myocardium to the fibroelastic sinuses takes place (Fig. 2.4). The fibrotic component, which represents the remaining 40% of the junction, includes the mitral-aortic continuity (between the left-coronary and non-coronary sinuses) and the membranous septum (between the non-coronary and the right-coronary sinuses) (Fig. 2.5). The dynamics of the ventriculo-arterial junction has been investigated in animal models. During ventricular filling and isovolumetric contraction, there is a circumferential expansion of both the ventriculo-arterial and sinutubular junction, while the entire aortic root elongates. The expansion at the ventriculo-arterial level is not symmetrical, being more accentuated along its muscular contour. Thus, the entire aortic root expands before the ejection and elongates, in order to accommodate the stroke volume. This expansion also reduces the area of leaflet coaptation, so that at the time of their opening, the leaflets are in apposition with each other with their free edge only. This mechanism is thought to decrease the friction between the leaflets during the valve opening. During the ejection phase, the ventriculo-arterial junction contracts, while the sinutubular junction

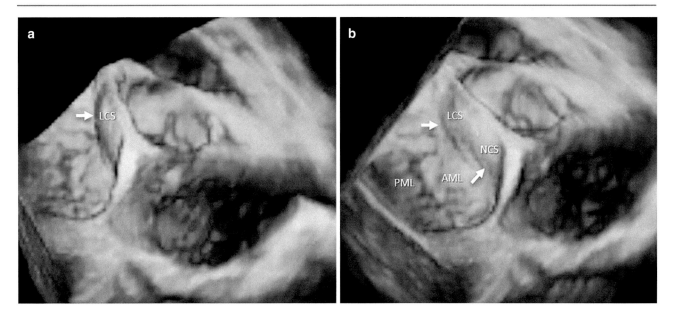

Fig. 2.3 (**a**) 3D TEE image from an oblique perspective, showing the left-coronary sinus (LCS) bulging into the atrial cavity. (**b**) Slight angulation of the same 3D data set showing both the LCS and non-coronary sinus (NCS) bulging into the left atrial cavity. *AML* anterior mitral leaflet, *PML* posterior mitral leaflet

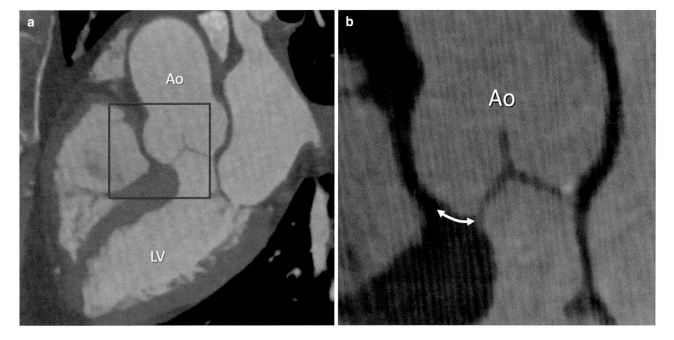

Fig. 2.4 (**a**) CT plane in long-axis orientation. (**b**) Magnified image from the red box in panel (**a**). The *double-headed arrow* marks the myocardium enclosed in the lower part of the aortic sinus. *Ao* aorta, *LV* left ventricle

continues to expand. Therefore, the shape of the aortic root changes into a truncated cone with the smaller diameter toward the ventricle. This "reversed" shape facilitates progression of the blood column towards the ascending aorta.

In humans, the so-called *fibrous skeleton* is limited to the right fibrous trigone and the membranous septum. The bundle of His runs immediately below the inferior margin of the membranous septum; the atrioventricular node is located in the so-called muscular atrioventricular septum (Fig. 2.6). Along with the fibrous adipose tissue of the atrioventricular groove, the fibrous skeleton separates the atrial and ventricular myocardium, ensuring that electrical signals from the atria reach the ventricles only through the atrioventricular node and the bundle of His. Moreover, it provides an anchor point between the valve leaflets and the muscular mass during contraction.

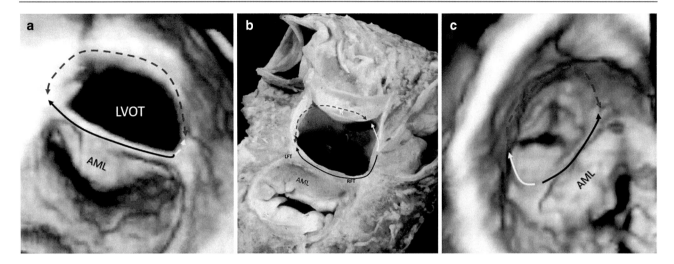

Fig. 2.5 The anatomic ventriculo-arterial junction from an overhead perspective (**a**) and a corresponding view of an anatomic specimen (**b**) following removal of the atrial walls, aortic sinuses, and the left-coronary and non-coronary leaflets. A ventricular perspective (**c**) delineates the mitral-aortic curtain (*black arrow*), the membranous septum

(*yellow arrow*) forming the fibrous part of the junction, and the muscular part of the junction (*red dotted arrow*). From both perspectives, the ellipsoid shape of the junction is observed. *AML* anterior mitral leaflet, *LFT* left fibrous trigone, *LVOT* left ventricular outflow tract, *R* right coronary leaflet, *RFT* right fibrous trigone

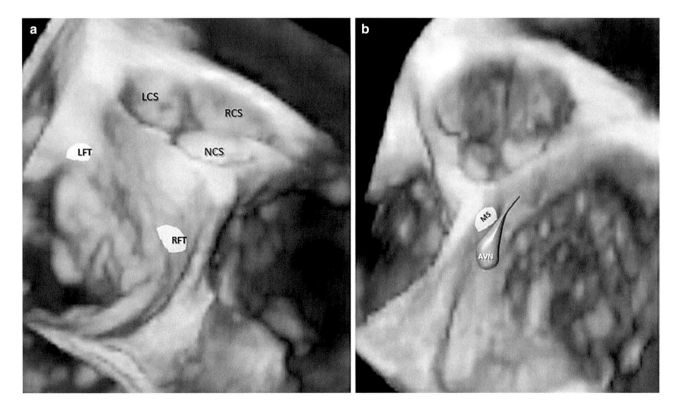

Fig. 2.6 (**a**) 3D TEE image showing the position of the fibrous trigones. (**b**) 3D TEE image acquired from another perspective, showing the position of the membranous septum (MS) and the atrioventricu-

lar node (AVN). *LCS* left-coronary sinus, *LFT* left fibrous trigone, *RCS* right-coronary sinus, *RFT* right fibrous trigone, *NCS* non-coronary sinus

The Crown-Shaped Annulus and the Interleaflet Triangles

As mentioned above, the hinge-line of the leaflets on the aortic wall has a crown-shaped configuration, with

the lowest part of the hinge-line lying slightly below the ventriculo-arterial junction (nadir) and the apical part joining the sinutubular junction (commissure) (Fig. 2.7). This arrangement guarantees aortic root flexibility, which would not be possible if the ring had a circular

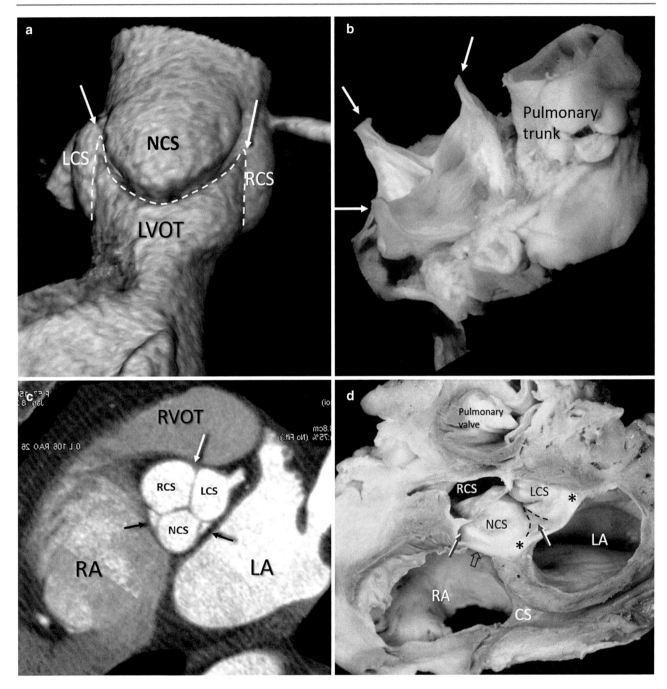

Fig. 2.7 (**a**) CT "electronic cast" image showing the posterior aspect of the aortic root with its "crown-shaped" insertion (*dotted line*). (**b**) Anatomic specimen after removal of the aortic sinuses and arterial wall, displaying the crown-shaped arrangement of the hinge line of the leaflets with the commissures (*arrows*) at the sinutubular junction. (**c**) Multiplanar CT reconstruction showing a short-axis slice of the aortic root with the three sinuses and the three interleaflet triangles (*arrows*).

(**d**) Anatomic section cut in similar plane to **c**, showing the mitral-aortic curtain (*between asterisks*), two of the interleaflet fibrous triangles (*red arrows*), and the membranous septum (*open arrow*). *CS* coronary sinus, *LA* left atrium, *LCS* left-coronary sinus, *NCS* non-coronary sinus, *RA* right atrium, *RCS* right-coronary sinus, *RVOT* right ventricular outflow tract

configuration. In fact, a fibrotic "ring-like" structure that would be robust and rigid enough to support the leaflets' insertion would probably result in an antegrade gradient comparable to the one measured across mechanical or biological prostheses (which feature a rigid, circular, unexpandable ring). Conversely, a crown-shaped configuration allows the ventriculo-arterial junction to expand and twist during systolic isovolumetric contraction and the early ejection phase, minimizing the transvalvular gradient.

This parabolic hinge-line has drawn attention to another component of the aortic root: the interleaflet triangles (Figs. 2.7 and 2.8). These three triangle-shaped fibrous structures are extensions of the left ventricular outflow tract. Rising from the plane of the "virtual annulus," they sit between the leaflets and reach the sinutubular junction, where the attachment of two adjacent leaflets creates the commissure. The triangle between the left-coronary and right-coronary sinuses is usually the smallest and separates the left ventricular outflow tract from the extracardiac space between the aortic root and the muscular infundibular sleeve of the right ventricle. The triangle between the left-coronary and non-coronary sinuses is made of fibrous tissue in continuity with the mitral-aortic fibrous curtain. This triangle is the largest and separates the left ventricular cavity from the transverse pericardial sinus. In small aortic roots, the mitral-aortic continuity and the corresponding fibrous interleaflet triangle is the site where surgery for aortic annulus enlargement is performed, in order to accommodate larger aortic valve prostheses. The triangle between the non-coronary and

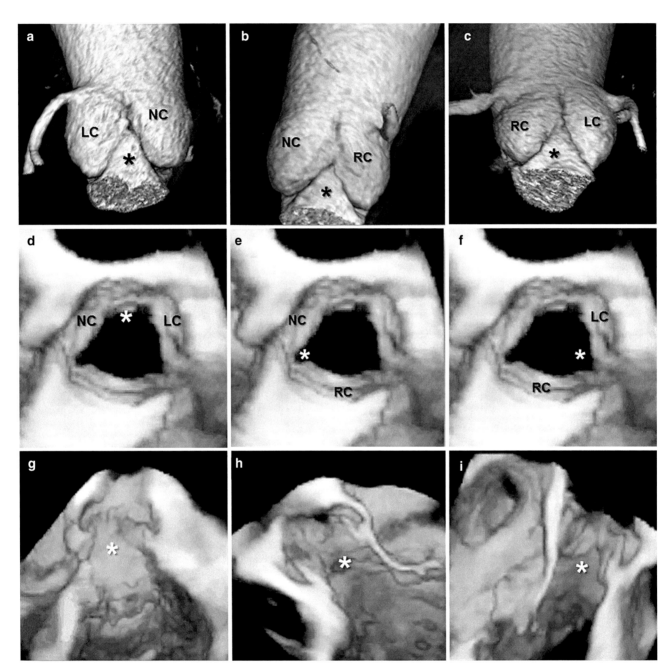

Fig. 2.8 (a–c) Electronic cast of the aortic root showing the three interleaflet triangles (asterisks). (d–f) 3D TEE from an aortic perspective. The positions of the interleaflet triangles are marked by the asterisks. (g–i) 3D TEE longitudinal sections of the aortic root showing the three interleaflet triangles "en face" (asterisks)

right-coronary sinuses adjoins the membranous septum, the site of the atrioventricular conduction bundle (*see* Figs. 2.6 and 2.7). Interestingly, all interleaflet triangles, though considered part of the aortic root, are extensions of the left ventricular outflow tract and therefore are subject to ventricular pressures. Thus, the interleaflet fibrous triangles, together with the ventricular surfaces, of the semilunar leaflets, mark the hemodynamic ventriculo-arterial junction.

The Sinuses of Valsalva

Behind each leaflet, the aortic wall bulges outward and creates the sinuses of Valsalva, which occupy the greater part of the aortic root. In a normal person, the three sinuses of Valsalva are named according to the origin of the coronary arteries. These pouch-like enclosures of different sizes extend distally up to the sinutubular junction, with the non-coronary sinus being the largest and the left-coronary sinus being the smallest. Histologically, the wall of the sinuses is made of collagen and elastic tissue and is thinner than the wall of the ascending aorta. The collagen fibers are more packed at the base of the sinuses, with a progressive increase in elastic lamellae progressing towards the sinutubular junction.

The main function of the sinuses is to preserve the integrity of the aortic leaflets, which open and close an average of 70 times per minute, for a mean total of three billion times during a lifetime. When closed, they withstand a pressure difference of 100 mmHg. This huge workload would in theory cause early leaflet degeneration if not for the protection by the aortic sinuses. In systole, their shape generates eddy currents between the leaflets and the aortic wall. Over the past three decades, the role of these eddy currents (first hypothesized by Leonardo da Vinci) has been confirmed by experiments and sophisticated valve models. Recently, it has been beautifully visualized with new 4D flow imaging obtained with cardiac magnetic resonance.

The eddy currents depend on the shape of the sinuses and on the narrowed sinutubular junction. The peripheral layers of the laminar flow generated during systole are limited by sinutubular junction narrowing and therefore are forced into a back flow directed towards the space between the leaflets and the sinuses. There, they promote a slow inward motion of the aortic valve leaflets, which start to approximate during late systole, so that the aortic valve is almost closed before forward systolic flow is complete. Therefore, when blood flow reverses in early diastole, the distance between the valve leaflets is minimal (Figs. 2.9 and 2.10). This phenomenon at low closing speed and minimal hemodynamic stress allows complete valve closure and prevents any volume leakage at closing.

The compliance of the sinuses (*i.e.*, the ability to distend under pressure) is another relevant characteristic that allows cyclical changes of the shape of the sinuses. An anatomical cross-section in the middle of the body of the sinuses reveals that the sinuses expand outward in diastole, assuming a three-lobed arrangement. This diastolic configuration splits the aortic root into three almost-circular subunits formed by the sinus and the corresponding leaflet. The "radius of curvature" of the three circumferences is smaller than the aortic root radius in systole. According to Laplace's law, the stress due to diastolic pressure is therefore reduced and shared in a single subunit between the sinuses and the leaflets. In valve-sparing aortic surgery, the maintenance or re-creation of the sinuses of Valsalva has been shown to effectively re-create the physiological vortices in the sinuses, so it may be beneficial in terms of normal leaflet movement and valve durability. Far from being inert flaps of tissue, the leaflets feature several types of valve interstitial cells (VICs), which continuously remodel the extracellular matrix by repairing functional damage, as discussed below.

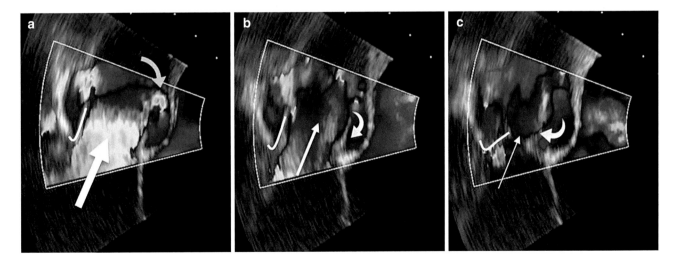

Fig. 2.9 2D TEE color Doppler imaging showing the effect of "eddy currents" (*curved arrows*), in early (**a**), mid (**b**), and late (**c**) systole

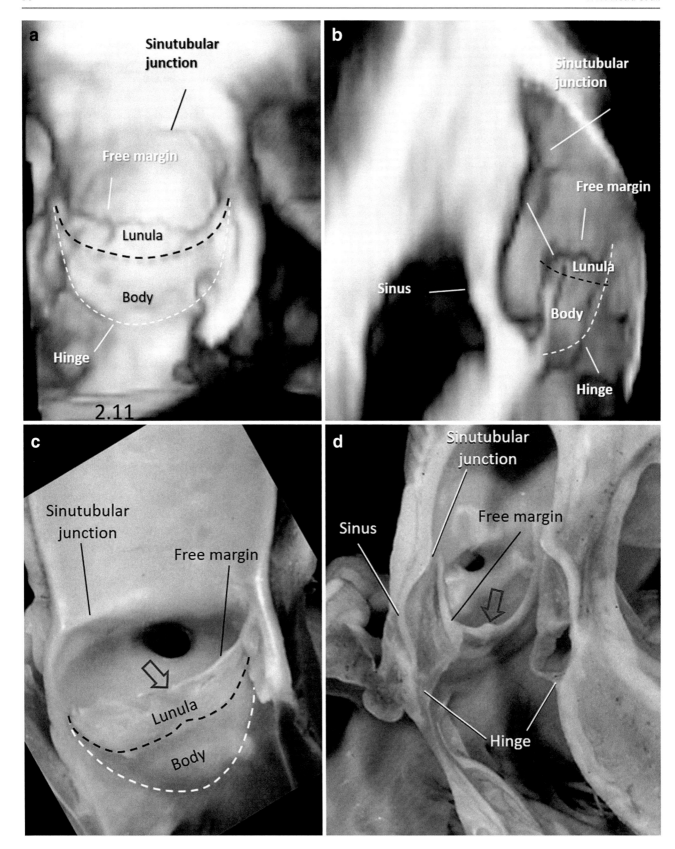

Fig. 2.10 3D TEE images showing the aortic leaflet "en face" (**a**) and in longitudinal perspective (**b**). The *black dotted line* outlines the inferior border of the lunula, while the *white dotted line* represents the hinge. The sinutubular junction appears on the internal surface of the root. The spatial resolution power of echocardiography does not allow for visualization of the nodule of Arantius. On the corresponding anatomical preparations (**c**) and (**d**), the *blue open arrows* indicate the nodule of Arantius on the free edge of the leaflets

The Leaflets

The aortic leaflets represent the "central piece" or the "working component" of the aortic root. The normal aortic root has three leaflets with slight differences in size and shape: the non-coronary leaflet is usually the largest, and the left coronary leaflet is the smallest. As described above, each leaflet has a parabolic hinge line (extending from the basal attachment with the left ventricular outflow tract to the sinutubular junction), a body, and an area of apposition, also known as the *lunula*. The lunula comprises approximately 30% of the leaflet total area. In elderly individuals, the lunula may be jagged or fissured, but this characteristic does not affect the valve competence, as these irregularities usually lie above the coaptation surface. In the middle of the lunula, at the free margin, there is a thickened nodule called the *nodule of Arantius* (Fig. 2.10). During diastole, each leaflet, together with the corresponding sinus, takes the appearance of a bird's nest. The insertion line of the leaflet is approximately 1.5 times longer than the length of the free margin, and the height (base to margin) ranges between 12 and 18 mm.

Leaflet microstructure: As discussed above, leaflets are not an inert layer of fibrous tissue; they are essentially a "living" structure. Histologically, they are composed of three layers: the *fibrosa*, the *spongiosa*, and the *ventricularis*. These layers are covered on both sides by a monocellular *endothelial layer*, which acts as a barrier limiting inflammatory cell infiltration and lipid accumulation. It also regulates permeability and cell adhesions, using paracrine signals. Under the endothelium of the aortic side, a thick fibrous layer or *fibrosa* is present, which mainly consists of collagen fibers with an "undulating" radial arrangement. Such "corrugated" fiber disposition allows for a higher degree of leaflet pliability, thus facilitating leaflet coaptation. During the cardiac cycle, the aortic leaflets change in size. Specifically, their area is about 50% larger in diastole than in systole. The fibrous lamina is therefore "stretched" in diastole and "wrinkled" in systole. On the ventricular side, elastic fibers predominate and form a layer called the *ventricularis*. The elastic lamina, by stretching in diastole and recoiling in systole, helps the fibrosa to maintain its "corrugated" configuration. Between the fibrosa and the ventricularis is a layer of loose connective tissue known as the *spongiosa*. The spongiosa is composed of extracellular matrix (mainly collagen fibers), complex glycoproteins, a network of nerve fibers and capillaries, and an array of different cell types, among which the most representative are the valvular interstitial cells (VICs). Each component confers specific physical properties to the extracellular matrix. *Elastin* allows for recoil after each deformation, and *glycoproteins* provide a "lubricant" characteristic, which reduces mechanical stress. VICs are essential in the processes of regeneration and damage repair. In other words, valve leaflets are able to self-repair, and the continuous renewal of all components is one of the secrets of their longevity.

The Sinutubular Junction and the Coronary Artery Ostia

The sinutubular junction (STJ) is the most distal part of the aortic root. It is a circular ridge that defines the origin of the ascending aorta; it is located between the aortic sinuses and the tubular segment of the ascending aorta (*see* Fig. 2.10). Anatomically, the STJ is more reminiscent of an "annulus" in the sense that the aortic wall, comprising mainly circumferentially aligned elastic lamellae, exhibits a mild waist that is accentuated by fibrous tissue at the attachments of the three commissures. Being a part of the aortic root, it contributes to aortic valve competence, so if the STJ is stretched, the result is aortic valve insufficiency. As mentioned above, the STJ plays a role in generating the eddy currents that help in leaflet closure.

The coronary ostia are usually located in the upper third of the sinuses of Valsalva, although individual hearts may show marked variability. Rarely, the coronary arteries arise above the STJ. At its origin, the right coronary artery takes off at a right angle from the aortic wall, whereas the left coronary artery originates at an acute angle. By using high-frequency transducers, small segments of the coronary arteries may be visualized with either TTE or TEE, and coronary flow can also be measured. Nevertheless, the best non-invasive imaging technique to visualize the coronary arteries remains CT imaging (Fig. 2.11).

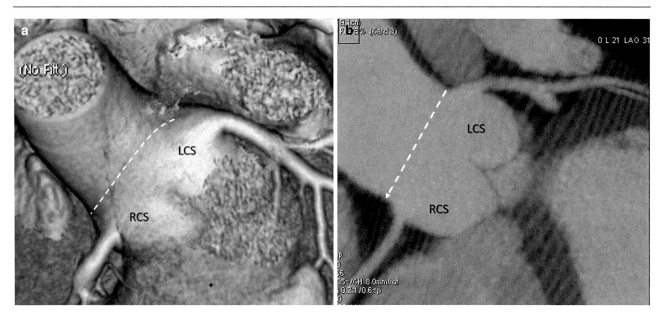

Fig. 2.11 CT volume rendering (**a**) and multiplanar reconstruction (**b**) showing the entire aortic root. The coronary ostia (*arrows*) are located in the upper third of the sinuses of Valsalva. The *dotted line* marks the sinutubular junction. *LCS* left-coronary sinus, *RCS* right-coronary sinus

Suggested Reading

Anderson RH. Clinical anatomy of the aortic root. Heart. 2000;84:670–3.

Anderson RH, Devine WA, Ho SY, Smith A, McKay R. The myth of the aortic annulus: the anatomy of the subaortic outflow tract. Ann Thorac Surg. 1991;52:640–6.

Davies RR, Gallo A, Coady MA, Tellides G, Botta DM, Burke B, et al. Novel measurement of relative aortic size predicts rupture of thoracic aortic aneurysms. Ann Thorac Surg. 2006;81:169–77.

Faletra FF, Nucifora G, Ho SY. Real-time 3-dimensional transesophageal echocardiography of the atrioventricular septal defect. Circ Cardiovasc Imaging. 2011;4:e7–9.

Ho SY. Structure and anatomy of the aortic root. Eur J Echocardiogr. 2009;10:i3–10.

McAlpine WA. Heart and coronary arteries. Berlin: Springer-Verlag; 1975. p. 9–26.

Piazza N, de Jaegere P, Schultz C, Becker AE, Serruys PW, Anderson RH. Anatomy of the aortic valvar complex and its implications for transcatheter implantation of the aortic valve. Circ Cardiovasc Interv. 2008;1:74–81.

Pisani G, Scaffa R, Ieropoli O, Dell'Amico EM, Maselli D, Morbiducci U, De Paulis R. Role of the sinuses of Valsalva on the opening of the aortic valve. J Thorac Cardiovasc Surg. 2013;145:999–1003.

Sutton JP, Ho SY, Anderson RH. The forgotten interleaflet triangles: a review of the surgical anatomy of the aortic valve. Ann Thorac Surg. 1995;59:419–27.

The Tricuspid Valve

Francesco F. Faletra, Laura A. Leo, Vera L. Paiocchi,
Stefanos Demertzis, Giovanni Pedrazzini, and Siew Yen Ho

Interest in the anatomy of the tricuspid valve has increased in the past two decades with the awareness that functional tricuspid regurgitation (FTR) is not an innocuous bystander of left-side heart disease but, on the contrary, is an insidious disease progressively leading to untreatable right heart failure and eventually to death. Most cases of severe tricuspid regurgitation are functional, due to right ventricular (RV) enlargement, annular dilatation, and leaflet tethering. Commonly, RV dilatation is secondary to left-side valvular diseases (mainly mitral valve stenosis or regurgitation), heart failure, and RV volume or pressure overload. Less frequently, severe FTR is the consequence of tricuspid annular dilatation due to isolated atrial enlargement caused by atrial fibrillation. Mild tricuspid regurgitation in the setting of a structurally normal tricuspid valve is a normal echocardiographic aspect.

A thorough knowledge of the anatomical architecture of the tricuspid valve and its spatial relationships with the surrounding structures may improve understanding of the process through which FTR occurs. In line with the other chapters, this chapter describes the normal anatomy of the tricuspid valve as revealed by computed tomography (CT), cardiac magnetic resonance (CMR), and two-dimensional (2D) and three-dimensional (3D) transthoracic echocardiography (TTE) and transesophageal echocardiography (TEE). The chapter concludes with a brief description of the patho-anatomy of FTR.

General Anatomy of the Tricuspid Valve

The tricuspid valve, positioned at the right atrio-ventricular junction, is the largest and the most apically positioned valve, oriented at approximately 45° to the sagittal plane. Although exposed to much lower systolic pressure, the global architecture of the tricuspid valve is surprisingly similar to that of the mitral valve. The complex valve apparatus usually consists of three leaflets, a circumferential hinge line where the leaflets are suspended, and a suspension system composed of chordae tendineae attached to papillary muscles or to the septum. In contrast to the mitral valve, however, where the architectural configuration is almost identical among different individuals, the tricuspid valve presents numerous anatomical variations in the number of leaflets and the arrangement of the papillary muscles. Furthermore, there is much discussion about the naming of the leaflets: Should a more attitudinal nomenclature be adopted? The septal leaflet is precisely just that, but the anterior leaflet is located more antero-superiorly and the posterior leaflet is more posterior-inferior. To enable team members to understand each other, we maintain the classic nomenclature of *septal, anterior*, and *posterior* for naming the leaflets, in keeping with common usage. Similar to Chap. 1, this chapter describes each component of the tricuspid valve apparatus separately.

The Tricuspid Annulus

The tricuspid annulus (TA), conceptualized as a discrete ring of dense, connective tissue from which the tricuspid leaflets are suspended, simply *does not exist*. Indeed, the right

F. F. Faletra (✉) · L. A. Leo · V. L. Paiocchi
Non-invasive Cardiovascular Imaging Department, Fondazione
Cardiocentro Ticino, Lugano, Switzerland
e-mail: Francesco.Faletra@cardiocentro.org;
lauraanna.leo@cardiocentro.org; vera.paiocchi@cardiocentro.org

S. Demertzis
Cardiac Surgery Department, Fondazione Cardiocentro Ticino,
Lugano, Switzerland
e-mail: stefanos.demertzis@cardiocentro.org

G. Pedrazzini
Cardiology Department, Fondazione Cardiocentro Ticino,
Lugano, Switzerland
e-mail: giovanni.pedrazzini@cardiocentro.org

S. Y. Ho
Royal Brompton Hospital, Sydney Street, London, UK
e-mail: yen.ho@imperial.ac.uk

© Springer Nature Switzerland AG 2020
F. F. Faletra et al. (eds.), *Atlas of Non-Invasive Imaging in Cardiac Anatomy*, https://doi.org/10.1007/978-3-030-35506-7_3

atrio-ventricular junction is made up of a juxtaposition of atrial and ventricular myocardium, separated by epicardial adipose tissue (EAT) of the atrio-ventricular groove and the hinge line of the tricuspid leaflets. However, for simplicity and consistency with the literature, however, we continue to name this part of the right atrio-ventricular junction as the *annulus*.

It is worth emphasizing that EAT is an integral part of the TA. This tissue of the atrio-ventricular groove, comprising adipocytes intermingled in a network of thin collagen and elastic fibers, extends up to the hinge line of the tricuspid leaflets. Except for the small septal area, where the hinge line of the septal leaflet intersects the central fibrous body and divides the membranous septum into two parts (see below),the EAT covers the entire anterior-lateral-posterior C-shaped groove and directly joins with the leaflets. The connective fibers of the leaflet fibrosa taper off into the fibro-elastic network of the EAT and the atrial and ventricular walls (Fig. 3.1a, b). This particular anatomical arrangement ensures excellent electrical insulation between the atrial and

Fig. 3.1 (**a**) Anatomical specimen cut in four-chamber plane. The epicardial adipose tissue (EAT) deeply penetrates (*dotted line*) in the atrioventricular groove up to the leaflet hinge line (*arrow*). (**b**) The corresponding histological section: the myocardium is stained red and fibrous tissue in the EAT is green. Adipose tissue appears as voids in the groove. The *arrow* points at the hinge line of the tricuspid leaflet. (**c**) 2D echocardiographic four-chamber view. (**d**) Magnified view of the area in the red box in panel (**c**). (**e**) CT scan, in four-chamber view. (**f**) Magnified view of the area in the red box in panel (**e**). Neither echocardiography nor CT is able to distinguish the EAT from surrounding structures. *RA* right atrium, *RCA* right coronary artery, *RV* right ventricle

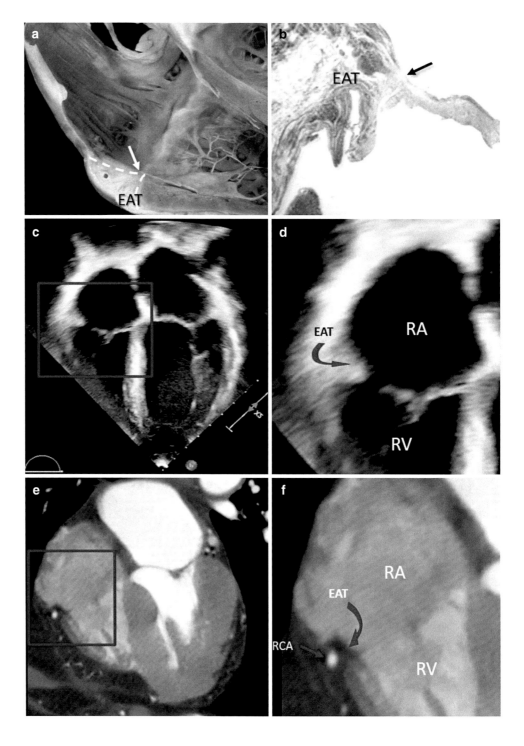

the ventricular myocardium, leaving the atrioventricular conduction system as the only myocardial tissue (specialized myocytes) crossing this barrier of insulation.

Echocardiography may potentially identify the EAT, which shows a characteristic hourglass appearance when it is extremely abundant, but although the atrioventricular groove contains relatively abundant EAT, the nearly identical acoustic impedance makes it rather difficult to differentiate between the EAT and the surrounding muscular tissue (Fig. 3.1c, d).CT scans can also differentiate the EAT from atrial and ventricular walls, because the EAT has a lower density than muscular tissue on x-ray and it is represented on CT imaging as a darker area. Despite the highest spatial resolution (voxel = 0.6 mm), however, the borders of the dark area corresponding to EAT and the borders of the surrounding muscular structures remain rather indistinct (Fig. 3.1e, f).

CMR balanced steady-state free precession (SSFP) sequences are ideal for a perfect delineation of the EAT in the atrio-ventricular groove and its extension up to the hinge line. In this sequence, in fact, blood and the adipose tissue produce a very high signal. Conversely, the signal originating from the muscular tissue is weak. The sequence therefore allows clear visualization of the EAT located in the atrioventricular groove (Fig. 3.2).

Surgical Aspect

For the surgeon, the hinge between leaflets and right atrium (RA) is clearly delineated by different colors: the wall of the right atrium is rather pale pink, whereas the leaflets have a yellowish-white color. Sutures are usually placed on the atrial wall 2 mm from the hinge line (to avoid damage to leaflets) and directed towards the ventricle to avoid the coronary artery.

From a surgical point of view, the TA can be described in terms of four segments: the aortic, anterior, posterior, and septal segments. This segmentation can be best understood by using 3D TEE technique, which allows the entire contour of the TA to be visualized in "en face" perspective. Figure 3.3 shows side-by-side the anatomic specimens (a, b) and the corresponding 3D TEE images (c, d) with the surgical segmentation of the TA (*dotted circles*) superimposed.

The *aortic segment*, adjacent to the aortic root, is the hinge line where the anterior part of the septal leaflet and the anterior leaflet are suspended; it includes the anteroseptal commissure. Identification of this segment in the operating room is of paramount relevance. Only a few millimeters (occupied by the transverse pericardial sinus) separate this segment from the aortic root (Fig. 3.3b, d).

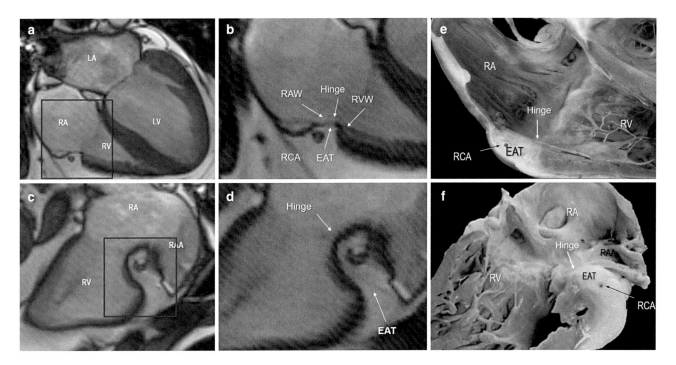

Fig. 3.2 Cardiac magnetic resonance (CMR) cine-sequence still frame obtained with steady-state free precession (SSFP) in four-chamber view (**a, b**) and in right ventricular inflow (**c, d**) view. The areas in the red box in the panels (**a**) and (**c**) are magnified in panels (**b**) and (**d**). (**b**) The image clearly shows the juxtaposition of the four components that form the tricuspid annulus: right atrial wall (RAW), right ventricular wall (RVW), epicardial adipose tissue (EAT), and the hinge line of the tricuspid leaflet. Image D especially shows how deeply the EAT penetrates into the atrioventricular groove. Corresponding cuts through anatomic specimens (**e, f**) show the hinge of the tricuspid valve leaflet (*white arrow*) and the deep excursion of the EAT into the right atrioventricular groove. *LA* left atrium, *LV* left ventricle, *RA* right atrium, *RAA* right atrial appendage, *RCA* right coronary artery, *RV* right ventricle

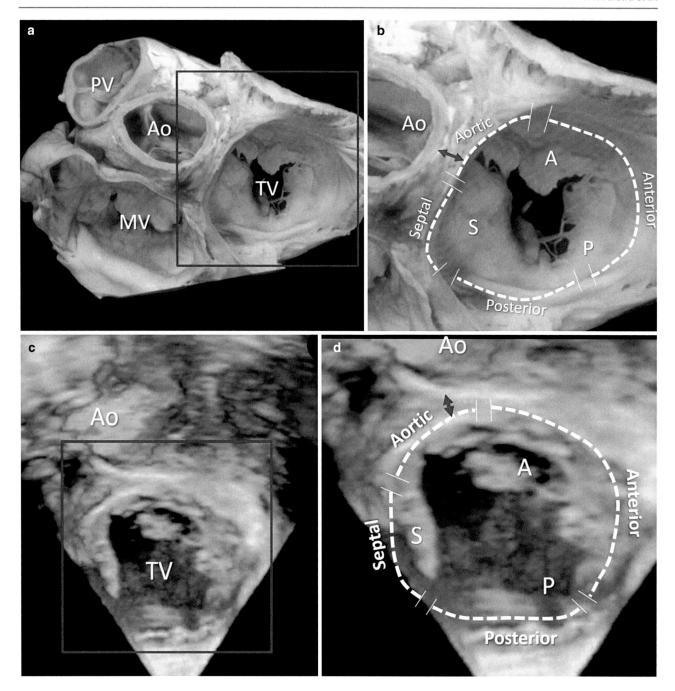

Fig. 3.3 (**a**) Anatomic specimen showing the base of the heart from the atrial perspective. (**b**) Magnified view of the area in the red box in panel (**a**), showing the surgical segmentation of the tricuspid annulus (TA). (**c**) 3D transesophageal echocardiography (TEE) image obtained from a transgastric view and oriented similar to the anatomic specimen in panel (**a**). (**d**) Magnified view of the area in the red box in panel (**c**), showing the surgical segmentation. The *double-headed red arrow* in panels (**b**) and (**d**) demonstrates the distance between the anterior segment of the TA and the aortic root. *A* anterior leaflet, *Ao* aorta, *MV* mitral valve, *P* posterior leaflet, *PV* pulmonary valve, *S* septal leaflet, *TV* tricuspid valve

During surgical valve repair or replacement with a prosthesis, imprecise suturing may damage the aortic leaflet or the right-coronary aortic sinus. Moreover, because of the strict anatomical proximity, large aneurysms or dilatation of the aortic root may alter the geometry of the TA, causing tricuspid regurgitation. Similarly, endocarditis or abscesses of the posterior area of the aortic root may invade the tricuspid valve.

The *anterior* and *posterior segments* of the TA are related to the free wall of the right ventricle. As described above, because of the absence of any rigid supporting ring, the TA tends to lengthen and enlarge along these segments. Conversely, the *septal segment*, being firmly attached to the membranous septum and reinforced by the right fibrous trigone in the vicinity of the antero-septal commissure, is relatively spared from annular dilatation, but the atrioventricular

Fig. 3.4 Anatomic specimen (**a**) and 3D TEE (**b**) in similar orientation, with the position of the atrioventricular node (AVN), the membranous septum (MS), and His bundle superimposed. The *yellow dotted line* marks the line for placement of surgical sutures. Tricuspid surgical rings are manufactured without the septal segment to avoid injuring the atrioventricular conduction system. (**c**) View of the septal surface of a heart specimen with the tricuspid valve opened to show the nonlinear hinge line (*blue broken line*) of the septal leaflet (S) in situ with its most apical attachment (*blue arrow*) and highest attachment (*open arrow*). The antero-septal (AS) and postero-septal (PS) commissures (comm) are indicated. Note the additional scallop (*asterisk*) in the posterior leaflet (P). (**d**) This enlargement highlights the membranous septum (*red broken line*) crossed by the hinge line. Leaflet tissue partially covers the interventricular component of the membranous septum, and there is a gap (*triangle*), not uncommonly seen in normal hearts. The antero-septal commissure is supported by a diminutive medial papillary muscle in this heart (*white arrow*). Thus, although a large portion of the septal leaflet has attachments to the septum (*small arrows*), a small portion is away from the septum. *A* anterior leaflet, *APM* anterior papillary muscle, *AVN* AV node and His, *CS* coronary sinus, *LA* left atrium, *RA* right atrium

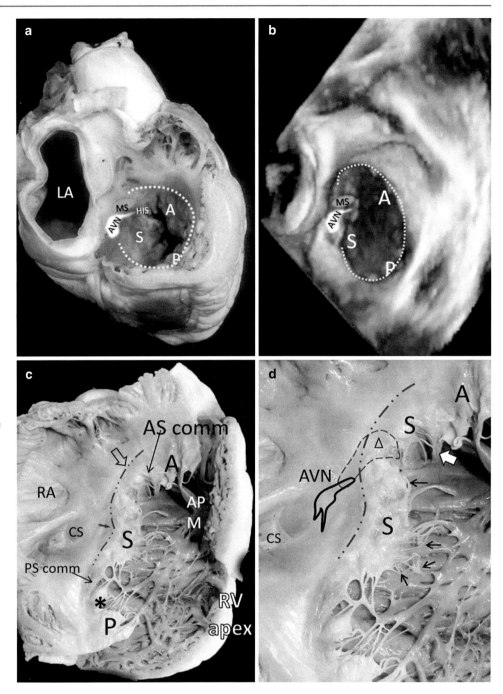

conduction system is located within the septal segment. In consideration of this fact, surgical rings are designed as "incomplete" rings, missing the septal segment, to avoid injuring the conduction system when placing sutures to secure the ring (Fig. 3.4).

Shape and Motion of the Tricuspid Annulus

The TA is almost oval (though in diastole it tends to be grossly circular). Similar to the mitral annulus but less accentuated, the shape of TA is not planar but roughly resembles a "saddle" configuration with two superiorly displaced regions corresponding to the anterior-septal and posterior-lateral segments and two regions displaced inferiorly, corresponding to the anterior-lateral and posterior-septal segments (near the ostium of the coronary sinus). This non-planar configuration is a consequence of several factors: the bulging of the right outflow tract, the undulating course of the anterior and posterior segments, and the position of the septal segment, which is attached lower, closer to the apex. Indeed, anatomic specimens clearly demonstrate the nonlinear hinge line of the septal leaflet. It is undulating, being most apical at a point close to the mid-portion of the leaflet's hinge and ascending toward the anterior-septal segment, peaking at the antero-septal commissure (Fig. 3.4c, d). The complex non planarity of TA requires a 3D imaging modality to assess its real size. Accordingly, the most recent data on TA size in healthy individuals are derived from 3D echocardiography (which showed a mean maximal circumference of 12 ± 1 cm and a mean area of 11 ± 2 cm^2) or from CT (which showed a maximum diastolic area of 10.7 ± 2.2 cm^2). Notably, the 3D measurements are smaller than those made on CT, probably because of differences in spatial resolution, which is higher with CT (isotropic voxel = 0.6 mm) than with 3D (anisotro-

pic voxel >1 mm). Interestingly, although in the literature these measurements refer to the TA, in reality they were taken on the hinge line of the tricuspid leaflets.

The TA has two fundamental motions: a sphincteric contraction and an excursion towards the apex. The *sphincteric motion* occurs because the anterior and posterior leaflets are attached directly on right ventricular myocardium and follow its systolic contraction. TA size (area, perimeter, and dimensions) progressively decrease during systole, reaching a minimum size in late systole and a maximum size in late diastole, after atrial contraction (Fig. 3.5a, b). The TA con-

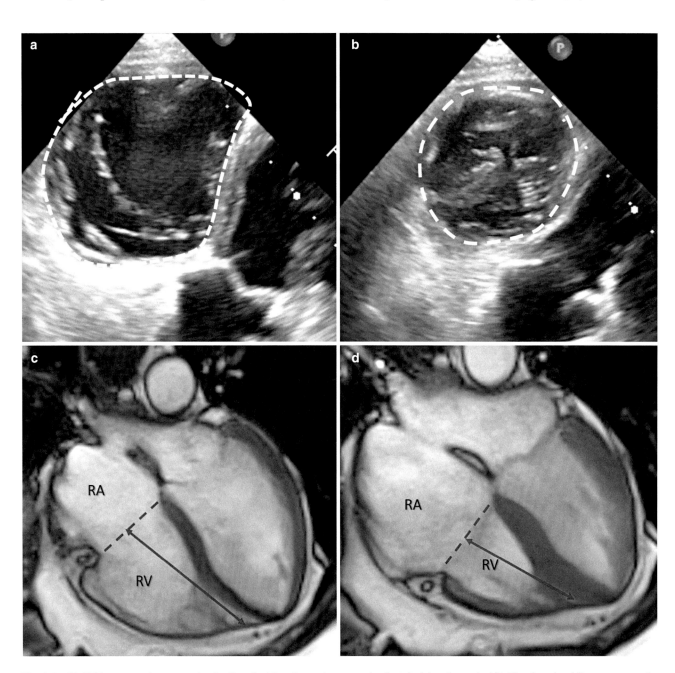

Fig. 3.5 2D TEE transgastric perspective in diastole (**a**) and systole (**b**), clearly showing the reduction in size of the TA (*broken line*). Similarly, CMR balanced steady-state free precession (SSFP) sequences using a four-chamber cut show the displacement of the TA towards the apex in diastole (**c**) and systole (**d**). The *dotted red line* represents the plane of the TA and the *double-headed arrow* shows the distance between the plane and the apex of the right ventricle (RV). *RA* right atrium

tracts 20% in dimensions and perimeter and 30% in area. Interestingly, in long-lasting, severe FTR, the TA becomes larger and more planar, losing its sphincteric action.

It is worth clarifying here the difference between the mitral annulus (MA) and the TA. The anterior segment of the MA is anchored symmetrically to the two fibrous trigones, and the posterior segment is made up of a fibrous (though incomplete) support. Conversely, the septal TA is firmly anchored at just one point, the membranous septum with right fibrous trigone (central fibrous body). The remaining antero-lateral-posterior contour consists of the hinge line of the leaflets attached to muscular and adipose tissue. Thus the sphincteric contraction of the MA is more regular, and the saddle-shaped configuration becomes more accentuated in systole, whereas the sphincteric contraction of the tricuspid valve is much more complex; it assumes a kind of "wave" motion depending on different degrees of contraction of the four segments and the rotation and translation of the atrio-ventricular junction.

The TA *excursion towards the apex* is due to the longitudinal shortening of the right ventricle. Because the part of the pericardial sac holding the apex of the heart is firmly anchored to the diaphragm through dense connective tissue bands, the systolic longitudinal contraction of the right ventricle causes a descent of the atrio-ventricular plane. 3DTEE and CMR may clearly show annular dynamics (Fig. 3.5c, d). In the normal individual, the tricuspid annular plane systolic excursion (TAPSE), measured by 2D TTE in four-chamber view, must be greater than 16 mm.

The Right Coronary Artery

Technically, the right coronary artery (RCA) is not part of the TA, but because of its proximity to the annulus and the potential complications that can occur during surgical and percutaneous transcatheter tricuspid valve repair, a brief description of the RCA course and its anatomical relationship with the TA is a useful adjunct to this chapter.

With the exception of the septal portion, the RCA runs within the atrioventricular groove encircling the entire parietal attachment of the tricuspid leaflets. The course of the RCA within the atrioventricular groove is undulating, and the distance between the RCA and the TA is variable. Several pathological and CT studies confirm the tendency of the RCA to run relatively further away from the TA in its anterior aspect (up to 20 mm away) and closer to the TA in its posterior aspect (less than 5 mm away).

The precise position in each segment between the RCA and the hinge line of leaflets is crucial information for both cardiac surgeons and interventional cardiologists. Direct injury by acute entrapment of the RCA by surgical sutures applied for ring fixation or RCA damage caused by annulus plication are rare but potentially life-threatening complications, which present as cardiogenic shock (due to acute RV failure) or electrical instability.

These complications are most likely in DeVega annuloplasty or if the expected anatomic distances between the RCA and TA are greatly altered by a very large TA. Impingement of the artery by pledgets or an anchoring system during tricuspid valve transcatheter annuloplasty is also a rare but potentially serious complication. There is no doubt that CT is the best imaging modality to visualize the particular anatomical relationship between the RCA and TA (Fig. 3.6a). In some cases, the anterior aspect of the RCA can be seen with 2D TEE transgastric short-axis view (Fig. 3.6b).

Leaflets

In the classic anatomy books and journals, the tricuspid valve traditionally has been described as having three leaflets (anterior, posterior, and septal) separated by three main indentations. The *anterior leaflet* is the largest, the most mobile, and has a semicircular shape. The hinge line of the leaflet extends from the antero-septal commissure to the antero-posterior commissure. Given its size, the anterior leaflet contributes the most to the competency of the valve. The *posterior leaflet* is smaller than the anterior, has a trapezoidal shape, and is attached to the posterior segment of the annulus. Finally, the *septal leaflet* is the smallest, is roughly rectangular, and is attached to the septal segment of the annulus. Anatomically, apart from being nonlinear, the antero-superior part of the hinge line of the septal leaflet crosses the thinnest part of the cardiac septum, which is composed of fibrous tissue and is termed the *membranous septum* (*see* Fig. 3.4c, d). Because the tricuspid valve hinge line is more apically located than that of the mitral valve, one portion of the membranous septum separates the right atrium from the left ventricular outflow tract while the adjoining portion separates the two ventricles. Thus, the membranous septum has an atrioventricular and an interventricular component (*see* Chap. 4). The atrioventricular part adjoins the right fibrous trigone of the mitral-aortic curtain, forming the central fibrous body. This is an important landmark for the location of the atrioventricular conduction bundle of His. Furthermore, the part of the septal leaflet at the membranous septum may take various morphologies (such as a small scallop or a bubble), or it may be partially or totally deficient, thereby leaving a gap in the closure line (*see* Fig. 3.4d).

The leaflets are separated by deep incisures called *commissures* at three locations: antero-septal, antero-posterior, and postero-septal. These commissures divide the valvular tissue into three main leaflets. Similar to the mitral valve, the three commissures do not reach to the hinge line. Thus, from a strictly anatomical point of view, the basal part of the leaflets toward the hinge line is a continuous veil of valvular tissue. The commissural tissue may be a simple strip or may assume the form of a small commissural scallop. Characteristic fan-like chordae are attached to the free edges. Each leaflet can be roughly divided in three zones: a basal zone of a few

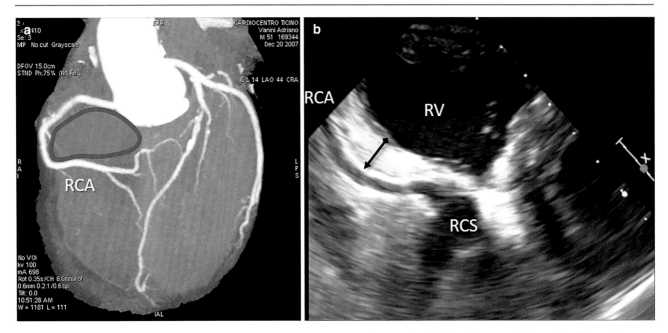

Fig. 3.6 (a) Maximum-intensity projection shows the RCA encircling the annulus of the tricuspid valve (*blue*). (b) 2D TEE (transgastric short-axis view) shows the anterior aspect of the course of the RCA. The *double-headed arrow* indicates the distance between the right ventricle (RV) and the RCA. *RCS* right-coronary aortic sinus

millimeters near the hinge line, a clear zone where the leaflet is thin and translucent, and toward the free edge is a rough zone, where chordae tendineae are attached on the underside. The rough zone corresponds on its atrial side to the coaptation area. The relatively large coaptation surface ensures that in systole there is nearly perfect competence of the valve.

As previously mentioned, the tricuspid valve morphology is hugely variable among individuals. This variability is particularly accentuated for the leaflets. Indeed, the entire tricuspid veil may be divided by indentations, which often do not conform to the classic scheme of three leaflets, as illustrated in Fig. 3.7. Some authors describe the tricuspid valve as having only two leaflets, septal and mural, an anatomic architecture that mirrors the mitral valve, where the antero-posterior commissure is diminished or lacking. Whereas the septal leaflet is hinged to the most robust and immobile part of the TA, the mural leaflet hangs down from the part of the TA that is related to the relatively mobile free wall. This part of the TA is characterized by significant changes in size and shape during the cardiac cycle, so the mural leaflet is required to have indentations to adapt the leaflet to the changeable annular area and to ensure opening of the leaflet, which otherwise would be restricted by a long intercommissural length. Indeed, quite often there is more than one indentation dividing the mural leaflet into up to six segments or scallops (Fig. 3.7).

Imaging Techniques

Both CT and CMR have several limitations in visualizing tricuspid leaflets. CT must use a dedicated acquisition protocol to optimally opacify the volume around the tricuspid leaflets.

Furthermore, visualization of leaflets' motion requires ECG-gated retrospective acquisition, which significantly increases radiation exposure. Finally, the frame rate (the number of images per second, up to 15 frames per second with the latest CT machines) is not optimal and is inferior to the other imaging techniques. When the space around the leaflets and in the right ventricle is opacified enough, however, the high spatial resolution of CT can visualize with unbeatable clarity the fine anatomic details of right ventricular structures such as chordae tendineae and papillary muscles. Because the leaflets are thin and fast-moving, they tend to be indistinct on images provided by CMR, which are often affected by blurring and ghost artifacts (Fig. 3.8).

Echocardiography is undoubtedly the first-line imaging technique for visualizing the tricuspid valve leaflets in real time. Both TTE and TEE can visualize the valve from several different views. It must be emphasized that 2D TTE and TEE use tomographic cuts that perpendicularly transect the leaflets, so their images represent only thin slices of leaflet tissue, and very few sections are able to transect the three leaflets simultaneously. In general, in normal individuals in whom the TA is elliptical, echocardiographic images of the tricuspid valve are of medium quality; images of the valve are unquestionably better in patients with a large TA.

Mid-esophageal 2D TEE should provide cross-sectional images of leaflets of higher quality than the equivalent cross sections of 2D TTE as are usual for the mitral valve, but mitral valve leaflets are relatively thick, are very close to the esophagus, and in systole are in a position almost perpendicular to the ultrasound beam. This fortunate combination of factors produces strong specular echoes that allow imaging from the mid-esophagus to produce, on average, images of the mitral

Fig. 3.7 (**a–d**) Anatomic specimens of the tricuspid valve showing the wide variability of leaflet morphology. The *asterisks* denote scallops. *S* septal leaflet

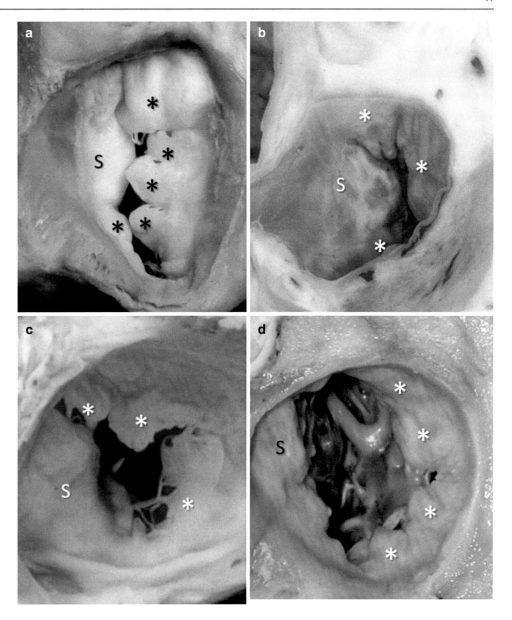

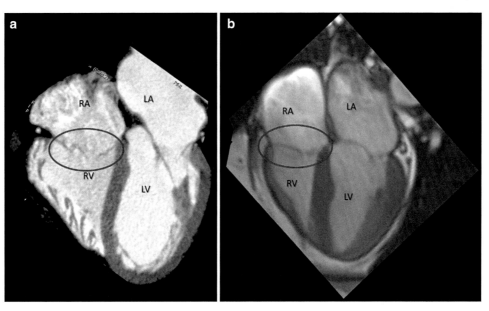

Fig. 3.8 Images of tricuspid leaflets (in *red ovals*) on CT scan (**a**) and CMR (**b**). *LA* left atrium, *LV* left ventricle, *RA* right atrium, *RV* right ventricle

valve of quality superior to the corresponding transthoracic views. On the other hand, the leaflets of the tricuspid valve are thinner than those of mitral valve, are further away from the mid-esophagus, and are in an oblique position with respect to the direction of the ultrasound beam. This *un*fortunate combination of factors often produces TEE images of tricuspid leaflets as a line with several artifactual interruptions (drop-out artifacts), most likely because the majority of echoes returning from the tricuspid leaflets are scattered and therefore are not strong enough to significantly contribute to the reconstruction of the final 2D image. The quality of transgastric TEE tricuspid valve images tends to be superior to mid-esophageal images, simply because the tip of the transducer is closer to the tricuspid valve.

Three-dimensional echocardiography has the potential to image the entire surface of the tricuspid leaflets in an "en face" perspective mimicking anatomic specimens. In patients with an optimal echocardiographic window, 3D TTE may provide diagnostic-quality images from the apical four-chamber view, but 3D TTE usually shows leaflets thicker than they really are, because of blurring or amplification artifacts. This phenomenon is less pronounced with 3D TEE. However, as for 2D TEE, 3D TEE suffers from drop-out artifacts due to the thinness of the leaflets and their obliquity with respect to the ultrasound beam. 3D TEE drop-out artifacts appear as small holes on the surface of leaflets. Figure 3.9 is a collage of tricuspid images obtained with 2D TTE and TEE and with 3D TEE.

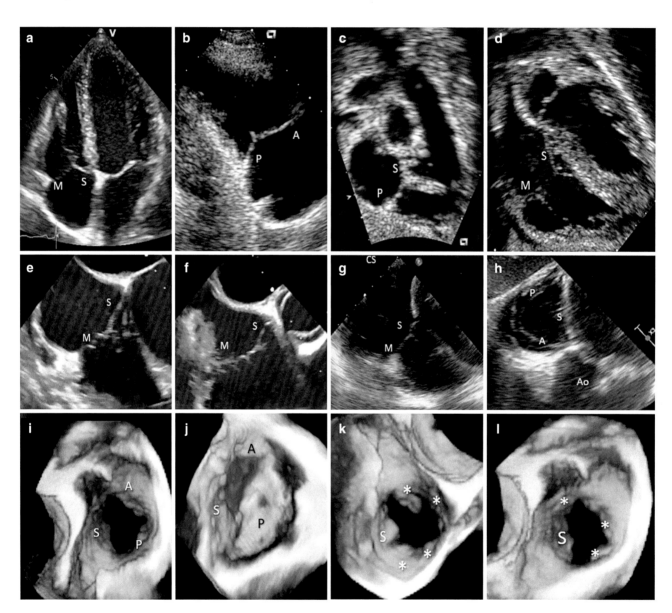

Fig. 3.9 A collage of tricuspid images obtained from 2DTTE (**a–d**), 2DTEE (**e–h**), and 3D TEE (**i–l**). In cross-sectional 2D echocardiography, the septal leaflet (S) is always recognizable because of its constant relationship with the septum and the aorta, but the anterior (A) and pos-terior (P) leaflets cannot be detected with certainty using cross-sectional planes, given the extreme variability of their size and number. In such a case, we prefer to label the posterior and anterior leaflets as mural (M) leaflet. (**k** and **l**) Scallops of mural leaflet are marked with asterisks

The Septal Leaflet

The septal leaflet deserves special attention. It is attached anteriorly to the membranous septum and posteriorly to the muscular atrioventricular septum (see Chap. 4). Typically, the posterior hinge line of the septal leaflet is apically displaced relative to the hinge line of the anterior mitral leaflet; this feature is always associated with the tricuspid valve, so it can be used to recognize a morphologically right ventricle even when the chamber is on the wrong side of the ventricular mass. The mean difference in levels (offset)

between the two hinge lines should not exceed 8–9 mm in the adult normal heart. An exaggerated offset could suggest Ebstein malformation. Unlike the other leaflets, the septal leaflet has multiple chordae tendineae attaching it directly to the interventricular septum, rendering it the least mobile of the leaflets. Notably, this septal attachment is probably the most constant feature of the tricuspid valve. Either TEE or CT scan can beautifully illustrate this anatomical peculiarity (Fig. 3.10). Furthermore, the septal leaflet extends antero-superiorly away from the membranous septum and the muscular ventricular septum because the commissure supporting

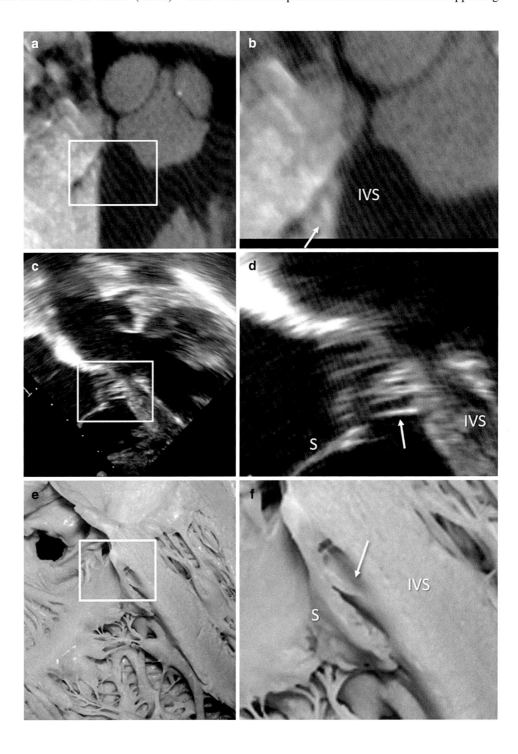

Fig. 3.10 CT scan (**a**, **b**), 2D TEE (**c**, **d**), and anatomic specimen (**e**, **f**) showing the septal leaflet (S) anchored with short chordae tendineae (*arrows*) directly on the interventricular septum (IVS). Panels (**b**), (**d**), and (**f**) are magnified views of the areas in the white rectangles in the other panels

the antero-septal commissure is attached to a small papillary muscle that arises from the posterior limb of the trabecular septomarginalis (TSM). This short part of the TA, no longer septal, relates instead to the aortic segment of the surgical view (*see* Fig. 3.3).

The septal leaflet is an integral part of the *atrioventricular junction*. In this characteristic area, the interatrial and interventricular septa join with the anterior leaflet of the mitral valve and the septal leaflet of the tricuspid valve. This region is discussed extensively in Chap. 4.

The Subvalvular Apparatus

The suspension apparatus comprises the chordae tendineae and papillary muscles (PMs). As for other tricuspid valve structures, PMs in the right ventricle are highly variable in number, position, and insertion of chordae, unlike the mitral valve. Classically, papillary muscles are described as being organized in three groups: anterior, posterior, and septal (or medial). The *anterior PM* is the largest and the most constant, being found in practically 100% of cases. It arises from the moderator band (MB) or the anterior wall at a level approximately one third of ventricular length from the apex. There may be one papillary muscle with two or three heads, or a group of smaller papillary muscles clustered together (Fig. 3.11). The chordae attach on the free margin and rough zones of the anterior and posterior leaflet and on the antero-posterior commissure. Particularly interesting is its anatomical relationship with the MB. Indeed, the MB originates from the body of the trabecula septomarginalis (TSM) and crosses the right ventricular cavity to insert into the RV anterior wall, from where the anterior papillary muscle takes origin. The "triad" of TSM, MB, and anterior PM forms a "U-shaped" structure that demarcates the inflow zone from the outflow zone of the right ventricle.

The posterior PM, arising from the posterior wall, is the least consistent. It is usually seen as separate, slender papillary muscles with chordae inserting to the free margin and rough zone. Short chordae attaching the basal part of the leaflet to the ventricular wall are seen in some hearts. As described previously, the antero-septal commissure is supported by a commissural chord attached to the medial (or septal) PM, also known as the muscle of Lancisi.This PM is small, singular or multiple, and arises from the TSM. The spatial distribution of chordae tendineae mimics its mitral counterpart, with marginal, secondary, and basal chordae. As mentioned above, the tricuspid valve characteristically has chordae tendineae directly arising from the interventricular septum to anchor the septal leaflet.

Pathoanatomy of Functional Tricuspid Regurgitation

Functional tricuspid regurgitation (FTR) has been neglected for a long time on the basis and assumption that it would simply disappear (or become irrelevant) at the time of mitral valve surgery. This long-held belief, derived from a study of Braunwald et al. published in 1967, had promoted in the past a conservative surgical attitude: Do not touch the valve. Now, however, evidence is clear that despite successful left-heart surgery with valve repair or replacement, more than half of patients with untreated FTR develop progressive valve dysfunction. Moreover, surgical series have demonstrated that any early reduction in tricuspid regurgitation following mitral surgery may be temporary; it may evolve over time to more severe FTR. On the other hand, despite the underlying tricuspid valve disease, patients with severe FTR after left-heart surgery remain mildly symptomatic, or even asymptomatic, for long periods, until overt right ventricular dysfunction occurs. As a consequence, repeat surgery for tricuspid valve repair is often reserved for patients who are older, with several comorbidities, and frequently are at the end stage of right heart failure. Not surprisingly, surgical mortality for an isolated reintervention of FTR repair/replacement performed years after left-heart surgery is higher than for any other single valve repair or replacement.

The European guidelines recommend tricuspid repair during left-heart surgery in the presence of severe FTR (class I; level of evidence C); moderate primary (organic) TR (IIa; C); and ≥mild TR with annular dilatation (≥40 mm) (IIa; C). The level "C" of evidence means that there is not unanimous consensus among experts, and this lack of strong evidence has probably contributed to the considerable under treatment of FTR. Thus, it is still unclear which criteria should be applied for tricuspid valve repair in patients undergoing mitral valve surgery. Although no longer forgotten, the tricuspid valve remains an "enigmatic" valve. We can prudently conclude that FTR is an insidious, unpredictable, and progressive disease leading to right heart failure and eventually to death if not treated at its early stages. A "prophylactic" repair of the tricuspid valve during left-side surgery is now an accepted surgical option, even for patients with moderate regurgitation, when annular dilatation is >40 mm. The German Transcatheter Mitral Valve Interventions (TRAMI) registry analyzed the prognostic impact of untreated FTR in patients undergoing percutaneous transcatheter procedures. The study found that patients with severe tricuspid regurgitation had elevated rates of atrial fibrillation, pulmonary hypertension, and residual mitral regurgitation, with decreased survival rates compared with patients without severe FTR. The negative impact that untreated FTR may have on these patients and the high mortality of a surgical option have

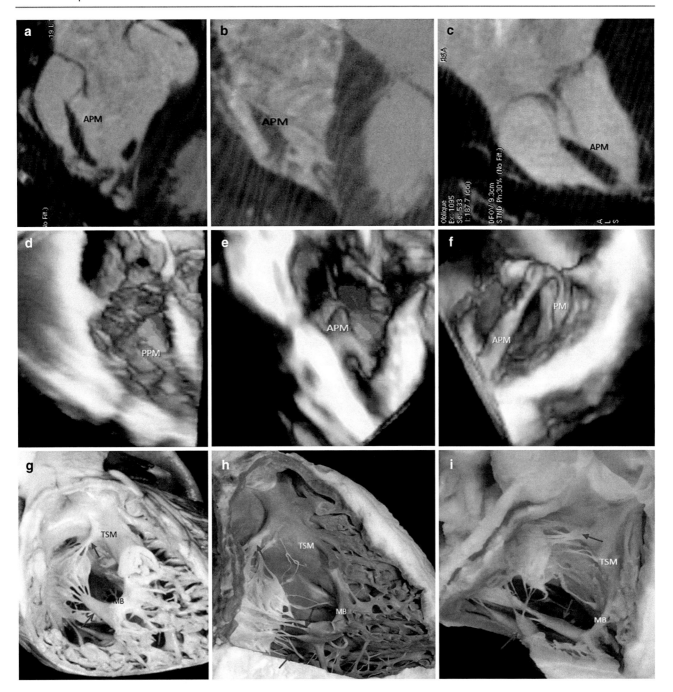

Fig. 3.11 (a–c) CT multiplanar reconstruction images showing the right anterior papillary muscle (APM). (d–f) 3D TEE showing the APM and posterior papillary muscle (PPM). (g–i) The anterior wall of the right ventricle has been removed from these three hearts to show some of the variations in the medial papillary muscle (*blue arrows*) and APM (*red arrows*). The trabecular septomarginalis (TSM), moderator band (MB), and APM form a U-shaped structure

highlighted the need to develop solutions for transcatheter tricuspid valve repair. Consequently, several catheter devices are currently under careful evaluation. There is still a lack of clinical data to support the efficacy of these transcatheter procedures, but transcatheter devices in selected nonsurgical patients may ultimately alleviate symptoms.

FTR represents the most frequent type of tricuspid valve regurgitation, accounting for 90% of all severe tricuspid valve regurgitation; other causes are far less common. Knowledge of normal tricuspid valve anatomy underpins a deeper understanding of the pathoanatomy of the tricuspid valve leading to FTR. As with functional mitral regurgita-

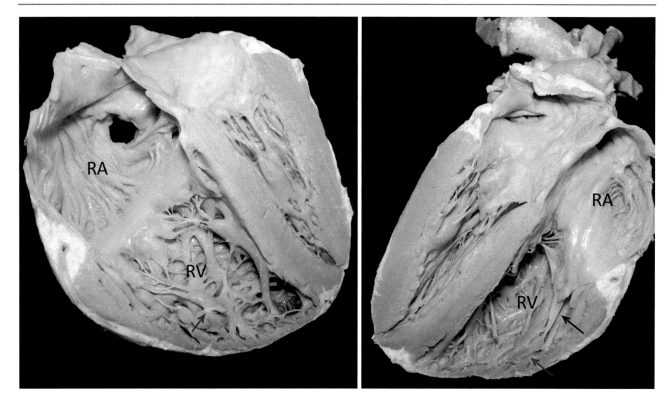

Fig. 3.12 Two halves of a heart specimen with remarkable dilatation of the right atrium (RA) and right ventricle (RV). The leaflet lengths from hinge line to free margin are too short to allow leaflet coaptation.

The anterior papillary muscle (*red arrow*) is displaced, and there is tethering of the anterior leaflet (*black arrow*)

tion, several mechanisms play a role in determining FTR, including annular dilatation, right atrial and right ventricular dilatation, displacement of papillary muscles, and tethering and tenting of leaflets (Fig. 3.12).

The peculiar anatomy of the tricuspid annulus results in asymmetric dilatation occurring mainly on the "free wall" hinge line, where the anterior and posterior leaflets are suspended. It is therefore not surprising that, in some patients with long-standing atrial fibrillation (AF), atrial remodeling may produce a direct effect on the annular hinge line, leading to FTR. As the annulus enlarges, posterior and anterior leaflets are pulled away from the septal leaflet and from each other, thereby diminishing the apposition zone between leaflets. In animal models, only a 40% annular dilatation may cause a regurgitant orifice with significant FTR. The susceptibility of the tricuspid valve to annular dilatation—and its prevalence compared with dilatation of the mitral annulus in patients with AF—is explained by the lack of accretions of strong fibrous tissue supporting the tricuspid annulus. The observation that some patients with long-standing AF do not have FTR is not yet well clarified. An individual tendency to develop right atrial remodeling or variations in leaflet size may explain these contradictory findings. The anterior leaf-

let, being the largest and the most mobile, may compensate for the annular dilatation, at least in the early stages. Patients with long-standing AF and FTR may not have enough leaflet tissue to adequately cover the increased orifice size. In cases of severe FTR, the surgical strategy includes either downsizing ring annuloplasty or leaflet augmentation.

More advanced FTR evokes a more complex interplay of factors such as annular, atrial, and ventricular enlargement. The RV dilatation determines displacement of PMs mainly towards anterior-lateral and apical directions. The chordae arising from the anterior PM tether the anterior leaflet, the adjacent segments of the anterior and septal leaflets, and the antero-posterior commissure, whereas chordae arising from the posterior PM tether the posterior leaflet and posterior-septal commissure. PM displacement leads to a loss of coaptation of the leaflets, which in turn worsens the FTR, with further RV enlargement resulting in a deleterious vicious circle. As in functional mitral regurgitation, leaflet tenting is the effect of tethering and a sign of severe tricuspid regurgitation. In this scenario, other pathologic changes occur: the tricuspid annulus loses its oval aspect and saddle-shaped configuration, becoming round and flat, and the sphincteric action diminishes. These pathological changes increase the distance between the hinge line and PMs, exacerbating the tethering on the leaflets. An effort to reorganize the complex mechanisms of FTR has been made by Dreyfus et al., who reclassified FTR into three stages roughly corresponding to the evolution of the disease:

- Stage 1: mild FTR, annular diameter <40 mm, normal leaflet apposition
- Stage 2: moderate FTR, leaflet coaptation limited at the edges
- Stage 3: severe FTR, annular diameter >40 mm, absent coaptation

These authors recommend medical therapy for stage 1, tricuspid annuloplasty for stage 2, and tricuspid annuloplasty plus leaflet augmentation for stage 3.

Suggested Reading

Beckmann A, Funkat AK, Lewandowski J, Frie M, Schiller W, Hekmat K, et al. Cardiac surgery in Germany during 2012: a report on behalf of the German Society for Thoracic and Cardiovascular Surgery. Thorac Cardiovasc Surg. 2014;62:5–17.

Braunwald NS, Ross J Jr, Morrow AG. Conservative management of tricuspid regurgitation in patients undergoing mitral valve replacement. Circulation. 1967;35(4 Suppl):I63–9.

Dean JW, Ho SY, Rowland E, Mann J, Anderson RH. Clinical anatomy of the atrioventricular junctions. J Am Coll Cardiol. 1994;24:1725–31.

Dreyfus GD, Martin RP, Chan KM, Dulguerov F, Alexandrescu C. Functional tricuspid regurgitation: a need to revise our understanding. J Am Coll Cardiol. 2015;65:2331–6.

Kilic A, Saha-Chaudhuri P, Rankin JS, Conte JV. Trends and outcomes of tricuspid valve surgery in North America: an analysis of more than 50,000 patients from the Society of Thoracic Surgeons database. Ann Thorac Surg. 2013;96:1546–52.

Nath J, Foster E, Heidenreich PA. Impact of tricuspid regurgitation on long-term survival. J Am Coll Cardiol. 2004;43:405–9.

Ohno Y, Attizzani GF, Capodanno D, Cannata S, Dipasqua F, Immé S, et al. Association of tricuspid regurgitation with clinical and echocardiographic outcomes after percutaneous mitral valve repair with the MitraClip System: 30-day and 12-month follow-up from the GRASP Registry. Eur Heart J Cardiovasc Imaging. 2014;15:1246–55.

Silver MD, Lam JH, Ranganathan N, Wigle ED. Morphology of the human tricuspid valve. Circulation. 1971;43:333–48.

Ueda A, McCarthy KP, Sanchez-Quintana D, Ho SY. Right atrial appendage and vestibule: further anatomic insights with implications for invasive electrophysiology. Europace. 2013;15:728–34.

Virmani R. The tricuspid valve. Mayo Clin Proc. 1988;63:943–6.

The Interatrial Septum, Septal Atrio-ventricular Junction, and Membranous Septum

4

Francesco F. Faletra and Siew Yen Ho

The Interatrial Septum

For full understanding of the relevance of a deep knowledge of the anatomy of the interatrial septum (IAS), this chapter begins with a brief description of the history of transseptal puncture (TSP) from its origin to the current day. Moreover, a brief clarification of interatrial septation in fetal life will help readers to better understand terms such as septum primum (SP) and septum secundum (SS), as well as adjectives such as "false" and "true" IAS.

A Brief History of Transseptal Puncture

Constantin Cope was an inspired cardiologist who, in 1959, first succeeded in catheterizing the left atrium by puncturing the IAS with the aim of assessing left atrial and left ventricular pressures. He used a self-made combination of a curved 7-Fr catheter over a needle. A few years later, Ross, Braunwald and Morrow provided the first exhaustive description of the transseptal left atrial puncture (TSP) technique. Finally, in 1962 Brockenbrough refined the procedure with several critical modifications of the transseptal needle. His catheter differs little from that used today.

At that time, TSP was an invaluable tool used for angiographic and hemodynamic assessment of valvular and congenital heart disease. Subsequently, the ability to register hemodynamic data with a less invasive Swan-Ganz catheter, the increasing use of retrograde left ventricular catheterization, and the introduction of Doppler echocardiography as a noninvasive tool for a reliable assessment of several hemodynamic parameters resulted in a decline in the use of this procedure. A resurgence in interest in TSP occurred in the 1980s and 1990s, with the introduction of percutaneous balloon mitral valvuloplasty and ablation of atrial fibrillation. More recently, the introduction of an impressive array of left-side percutaneous catheter-based interventions for structural heart disease led to the widespread adoption of TSP. Nowadays, TSP is probably the most widely used percutaneous technique, being the first step in all of the catheter-based procedures for the left side.

In the early days, the main concern of the pioneering interventionalists and electrophysiologists was to "safely" cross the IAS, preferably through the fossa ovalis (FO). At that time, the only guide to achieve this goal was fluoroscopic imaging aided by the tactile feedback of skilled operators. Although they were completely "blind" (as fluoroscopy does not allow visualization of the IAS), the TSP was performed safely in most cases, with a rate of complications less than 1%. Even today, expert electrophysiologists usually perform the TSP blindly, asking for transesophageal echocardiography (TEE) or intracardiac echocardiography (ICE) only in difficult cases, such as those with extreme rotation of the heart, lipomatous IAS, or previous transseptal puncture. However, the increasingly complex percutaneous procedures performed today necessitate "site-specific" TSP, for which TEE or ICE becomes an essential tool for providing a high degree of anatomic precision. For instance, in a mitral clip procedure, the TSP is the most important initial step. TSP in a suboptimal site may result in an inadequate and long procedure. As shown in Fig. 4.1, the correct site of the TSP to reach a regurgitant orifice located between A2 and P2 must be superior and posterior, but lateral or medial regurgitant orifices require punctures that are more superior-anterior or inferior-posterior, respectively, but always within the FO.

F. F. Faletra (✉)
Non-invasive Cardiovascular Imaging Department,
Fondazione Cardiocentro Ticino, Lugano, Switzerland
e-mail: Francesco.Faletra@cardiocentro.org

S. Y. Ho
Royal Brompton Hospital, Sydney Street, London, UK
e-mail: yen.ho@imperial.ac.uk

© Springer Nature Switzerland AG 2020
F. F. Faletra et al. (eds.), *Atlas of Non-Invasive Imaging in Cardiac Anatomy*, https://doi.org/10.1007/978-3-030-35506-7_4

Fig. 4.1 (**a** and **b**) Different
site-specific transseptal
punctures (TSPs) in a mitral
clip procedure, seen in 3D
transesophageal
echocardiography (TEE). If
the regurgitant orifice is
central (at A2-P2 level) the
interatrial septum should be
punctured high and posterior
(*red spot* and *red curved
arrow*). If the regurgitant
orifice is more lateral, the
interatrial septum should be
punctured more anterior and
superior (*yellow spot* and
yellow curved arrow). Finally,
if the regurgitant orifice is
more medial, the site of TSP
should be more posterior
(*grey spot* and *curved arrow*).
(**c** and **d**) The corresponding
anatomic specimens. *Ao* aorta,
CS coronary sinus, *FO* fossa
ovalis, *TV* tricuspid valve

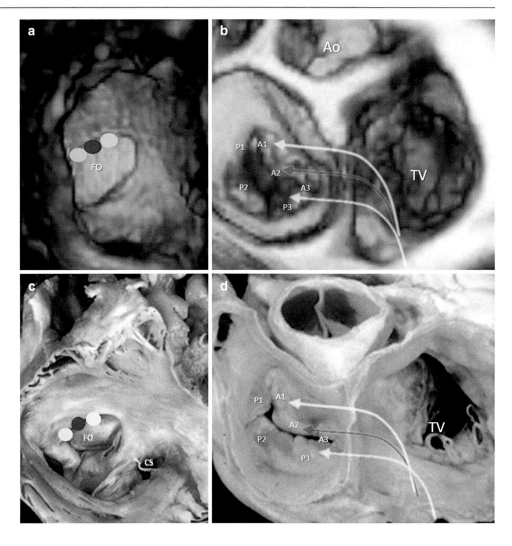

Septation of the Atria

During cardiac development, the appearance of the so-called
septum primum (SP) indicates the onset of atrial septation. It
begins as a thin crescent of tissues in the atrial roof.
Mesenchymal cells, derived from embryonic endocardium,
cover the free edge of the SP (mesenchymal cup). The SP
gradually advances into the primitive atrium, towards the
endocardial cushions. At the same time, the upper part breaks
down, forming a hole, the so-called ostium secundum (OS)
The OS allows blood flow through the primitive septation to
reach the left heart once the ostium primum (OP), the space
between the leading edge of the SP and the fused cushions, is
obliterated. Contemporaneously, a folding of the atrial wall,
the so-called septum secundum (SS), is formed to the right
side of the SP; it rises and extends anteriorly, superiorly, posteriorly and inferiorly to overlap the SP. Thus, seen from the
right atrial perspective, the SP becomes the floor of the oval-
shaped depression (fossa ovalis) bounded by the enfolded SS
rim. In fetal life, this septum works as a flap valve guiding
the blood flow from the right atrium to the left atrium through

the OS. After birth, when higher pressure in the left atrium
pushes the flap valve against the muscular rim, the OS closes.

There is a large amount of literature carefully describing
the anatomy of the IAS and the atrio-ventricular (AV) junction, mostly written by anatomists who illustrated their
descriptions with cadaveric specimens. These descriptions
remain the state-of-the-art for the heart anatomy, but today
noninvasive techniques such as cardiac magnetic resonance
(CMR) , two- and three-dimensional transesophageal echocardiography (2D/3D TEE), and CT scans allow us to see
exquisite anatomic details of cardiac structures in both two-
and three-dimensional formats. Interventional cardiologists
and electrophysiologists frequently use these noninvasive
techniques either before or during catheter-based structural
heart disease and electrophysiology procedures. Thus,
describing the normal anatomy of the IAS and the AV junction through these noninvasive imaging modalities has never
been more important for performing a safe and efficacious
TSP. This chapter provides a detailed description of the anatomy of the IAS as illustrated by these noninvasive imaging
techniques.

"True" Interatrial Septum

The medial wall of the left and right atria, when observed from both atrial perspectives, appears to be an extensive area, but this impression is deceptive. On the right atrial side, it seems to be bordered inferiorly by the orifice of the inferior vena cava (IVC) and superiorly by the superior vena caval (SVC) orifice; the anterior-inferior border is the hingeline of the tricuspid valve, and the bulging aortic non-coronary sinus marks the antero-superior border. On the left atrial side, the borders are perceived to be the right pulmonary veins posteriorly, the mitral hingeline inferiorly, and non-coronary aortic sinus antero-superiorly. CMR and CT are intrinsically three-dimensional modalities, but although they can reconstruct the "external" surface, they cannot illustrate the "internal" surfaces of the heart, which require substantially "cross-sectional" modalities. Conversely, 3D TEE has the unique ability of showing the surfaces of the IAS from both left-side and right-side perspectives with an accuracy comparable to anatomic specimens. For that reason, 3D TEE is probably the most appropriate modality to describe this area and its anatomical relationships (Fig. 4.2).

Historically the medial wall of both atria, formed by the embryonic SP and embryonic muscular SS, has been considered the partition interposed between the two atria—in other words, the IAS. But when anatomists describe the IAS as a wall interposed between the right and left atrial cavities, they refer to the fact that removal or puncturing of this area creates a communication directly between the two atria, not via extracardiac tissues or space. This anatomist's definition corresponds to the floor of the FO, which is nearly one fifth of

the abovementioned extensive area; only the FO, as delimited by the red circle in Fig. 4.2, is unquestionably the "true" septum.

The muscular area surrounding the posterior, superior, and inferior margins of the FO (known as the septum secundum [SS])actually does not separate the right from the left atrium without traversing through epicardial tissues. This area is an infolding of the atrial roof positioned between the orifice of the SVC and the right pulmonary vein. Removing or puncturing this region causes an exit from the cavities of the heart into epicardial fat or, worse still, into extracardiac space. Thus, although commonly referred as "septum secundum," this infolding is definitively not a proper "septum."

Correctly described in the nineteenth century by Waterston and known as Waterston's or Sondergaard's groove (or simply as the superior interatrial groove), this infolding contains epicardial adipose tissue and small vessels. Because of their tomographic nature, 2D and 3D TEE produce cross-sectional cuts that depict the FO as a thin membrane and the SS as a thicker, muscular septum. Both techniques usually fail to identify the adipose tissue inside the folding. Indeed, the similar acoustic impedance between muscular and adipose tissue and the fact that, in normal individuals, this infolding is usually almost virtual, make it very difficult to differentiate the small amount of adipose tissue from the two atrial walls (Fig. 4.3).

CT can identify adipose tissue inside the infolding; the adipose tissue appears darker because it has a lower density than the surrounding muscular tissue. Despite the high spatial resolution of the technique (voxel = 0.6 mm), however, the borders between adipose tissue and muscular atrial wall remain rather indistinct (Fig. 4.4a).

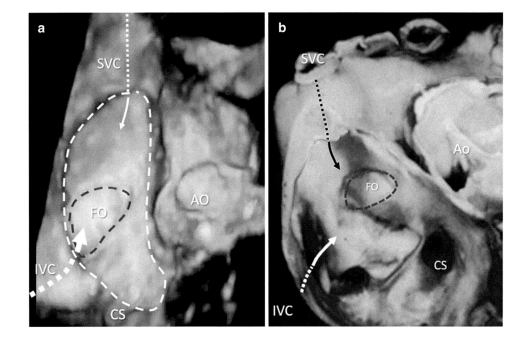

Fig. 4.2 (**a**) 3D TEE showing the extensive area (*white dotted circle*) observed from a right atrial perspective that at first sight seems a wall interposed between the two atria. The *red dotted circle* marks the boundaries of the fossa ovalis (FO) (see text). *Arrows* indicate the pathway of the superior vena cava (SVC) and inferior vena cava (IVC). (**b**) Corresponding anatomic specimen. *CS* coronary sinus, *AO* aorta

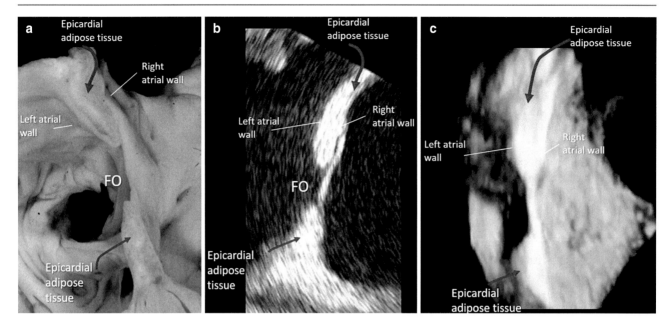

Fig. 4.3 (**a**) Anatomic specimen cross-sectional cut shows the infolding of atrial wall filled with epicardial adipose tissue, forming the septum secundum (see text). (**b** and **c**) Cross-sectional 2D and 3D TEE images of the interatrial septum (IAS). Both images fail to clearly illustrate this particular anatomic architecture

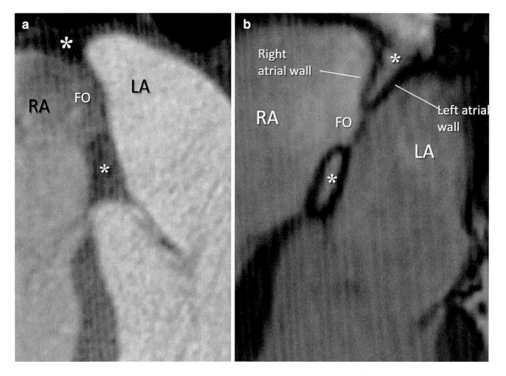

Fig. 4.4 (**a**) Cross section obtained with multiplanar CT. With this technique, the adipose tissue has a lower density than surrounding muscular walls and therefore it appears darker (*asterisks*). Despite the high spatial resolution of the technique (voxel = 0.6 mm), however, borders between adipose tissue and atrial wall remain rather indistinct. (**b**) Cardiac magnetic resonance (CMR) steady state free precession (SSFP) sequence. With this sequence, the muscular tissue produces weak signals and therefore appears darker than blood and adipose tissue, which produce stronger signals and so appear brighter. This difference allows a clear distinction between the atrial walls and the external adipose tissue (*asterisks*). *FO* fossa ovalis, *LA* left atrium, *RA* right atrium

Probably the best imaging modality to illustrate the complex architecture of IAS is CMR. CMR imaging of the septum maintains the same 2D format as CT and 2D TTE/TEE, but CMR allows a clear distinction between muscular and adipose tissue when a specific pulse sequence called steady state free precession (SSFP) is used. SSFP provides a high signal/noise ratio and optimal blood/myocardium contrast, which allows a precise definition of the endocardial borders. Furthermore, in this sequence, the strength of the signal orig-

inating from different tissues depends on the T1/T2 ratio. Both blood and adipose tissue have the same high T1/T2 ratio, so both tissues produce a very high signal. Conversely, muscular tissue has a low T1/T2 ratio, so the signal originating from this tissue is weak. The sequence therefore can clearly distinguish the adipose tissue located into the fold of the atrial walls (Fig. 4.4b).

In Fig. 4.5, panel (a) shows a CMR four-chamber view. A cut through the dotted line results in a cross-sectional slice

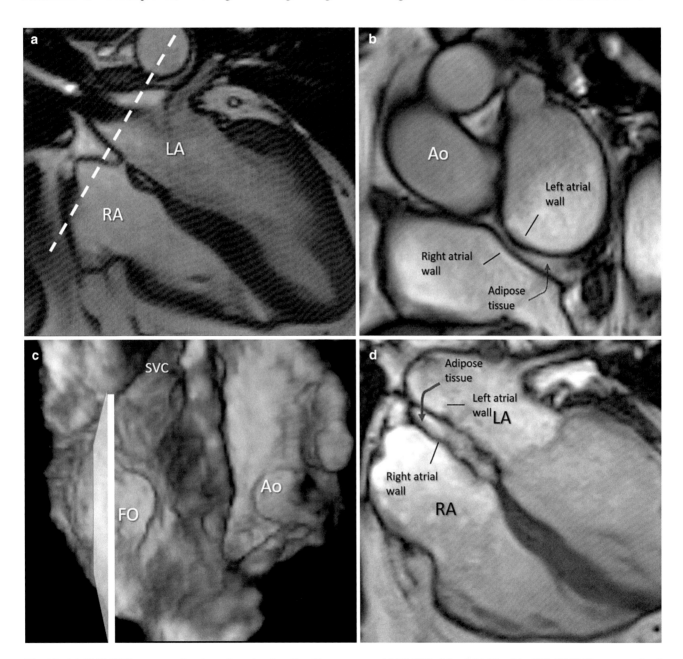

Fig. 4.5 (**a**) CMR SSFP sequence showing a four-chamber slice. From this image, it is clear that the superior part of the IAS is an infolding of the right and left atrial wall. (**b**) Cross-sectional slice through the dotted line of panel (**a**), passing through the atria and showing the three-layered appearance of the septum secundum. Removal or puncturing of this region opens the atrial wall to epicardial tissues or extracardiac

space. (**c**) 3D TEE of the right side of the IAS. (**d**) CMR cross-sectional slice through the superimposed white plane of panel (**c**). This slice shows that the infolding extends posteriorly and inferiorly, buttressing the inferior margin of the fossa ovalis (FO) and joining with the septal atrio-ventricular junction. *Ao* aorta, *LA* left atrium, *RA* right atrium, *SVC* superior vena cava

through the two atria, demonstrating clearly the three-layered structure of the SS formed by the right atrial wall, adipose layer, and left atrial wall (panel b). Similarly, a cross-sectional slice inferior to the FO shows the same "three-layered" aspect of the SS that extends posteriorly and inferiorly, buttressing the inferior margin of the FO and joining the septal AV junction (panels c and d).

The size of the FO may vary, depending on the extension of the in folding and on the atrial size (Fig. 4.6). Generally, the largest FOs are those with large atria. In some cases, stretching of the FO due to voluminous atria may create an atrial septal defect. The smallest FOs are those associated with abundant accumulation of adipose tissue in the infolding, the so-called lipomatous hypertrophy of the IAS.

Defining the size of the FO is important because the only site for the safest transseptal crossing is through the FO (Fig. 4.7a, b). Another area of interest is the superior-anterior region. This area abuts the transverse pericardial sinus and, through it, the aortic root, the most important structure close to the FO. Only a few millimeters separate the anterior-superior margin of the FO from the right atrial wall, which overlies the right-coronary aortic sinus anteriorly and the non-coronary aortic sinus posteriorly. The most feared complication during a "blind" crossing through the FO is puncture into the aortic root (Fig. 4.7c, d).

Misconceptions

Misinterpretation of the peculiar anatomy of the IAS has led to several misnomers. The first is *lipomatous hypertrophy of the IAS*, coined by Prior in 1964, which is incorrect for three reasons. Unlike lipoma, the lipomatous tissue of the IAS is not encapsulated. Moreover, the lipomatous "hypertrophy" is histologically characterized by an increased number of adipocytes (hyperplasia), not by an increased size of individual adipocytes (hypertrophy). Finally, this accumulation of adipocytes belongs to epicardial adipose tissue and fills the interatrial groove, so it is completely external to the IAS. CMR sequences may exquisitely define the external nature of this adipose tissue, and a careful inspection of this entity with 2D/3D TEE clearly shows that this tissue has the hourglass appearance characteristically defining the adipose tissue. Thus, *lipomatous hypertrophy of the IAS* should simply be called *abnormal accumulation of adipose tissue in the interatrial groove*. It is a benign entity, although a large amount of adipose tissue may obstruct the SVC inflow or cause distortion of the atrial walls, with consequent atrial arrhythmias.

Second, the subtypes of atrial septal defect (ASD), which include superior and inferior sinus venosus defects, ostium primum, and unroofed coronary sinus, are termed "interatrial septal communications," or ASD for short. But

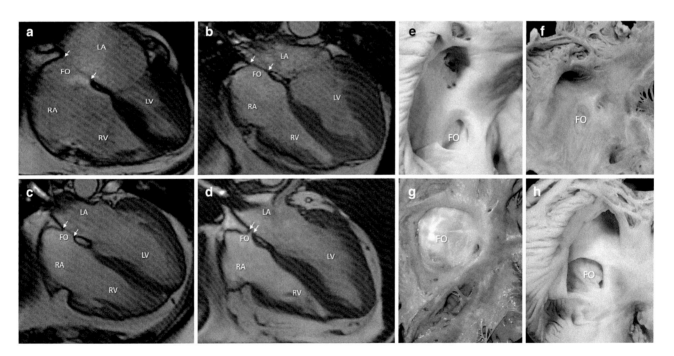

Fig. 4.6 (**a–d**) Cross-sectional images obtained with CMR sequences showing the different sizes of the fossa ovalis (FO). *Arrows* delimit the boundaries of the FO. (**e–h**) Right atrial view of anatomic specimens showing variations in sizes and morphologies of FO. *LA* left atrium, *LV* left ventricle, *RA* right atrium, *RV* right ventricle

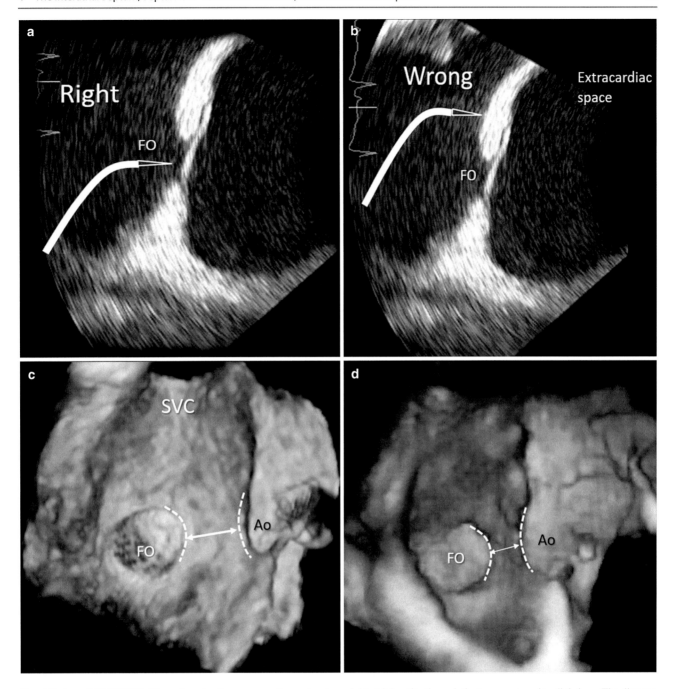

Fig. 4.7 (**a** and **b**) 2DTEE. The safest site for transseptal crossing is the fossa ovalis (FO). Puncturing the region called the septum secundum from within the right atrium produces an exit from the atrial cavities into epicardial tissues occupying the infolding and potentially into extracardiac space. (**c** and **d**) 3DTEE. The aortic root (Ao) abuts the right atrial cavity through the transverse pericardial sinus. The distance between the superior-anterior margin of the FO and the area where the aortic root abuts (*double-headed arrow*) is variable. The most feared complication during a blind crossing of the FO is puncture into the aortic root

the shunt between the atrial chambers in these subtypes occurs outside the confines of the true atrial septum. A more correct term would be "interatrial extra-septal communications" or simply "interatrial communications." A defect in the FO (so-called secundum ASD) is the only true ASD and can be treated percutaneously with implantation of a device. For large ASDs with a complete absence of the septum primum, the device directly embraces the infolding of the atrial wall.

Third, the old classification of a septal aneurysm as being "limited" to the FO or "involving the entire septum" does not make sense. It is inconceivable that the three-layered, fat-filled muscular sandwich that forms the SS could be involved in an aneurysmal formation. The septal aneurysm is *always* limited to the FO; it may be small or large according the size of the FO.

The Septal Pouch *Versus* Patent Foramen Ovale

The septal pouch is an anomaly that was first highlighted only about 2010. To understand it better, it is appropriate to review the anatomy of the patent foramen ovale (PFO). In fetal life, blood from the right atrium pushes the flap valve of the FO into the left atrium to allow flow through the ostium secundum. After birth, the flap valve (which is normally larger than the FO) is pushed back toward the muscular rim of the SS, thereby closing the ostium secundum. The valve normally becomes adherent to the rim around its entire margin, creating an intact septum and obliterating any possibility of interatrial shunts. Up to a quarter of the normal population, however, has a PFO, which is due to lack of adhesion at the valvular border of the ostium secundum, the free edge of the septum primum. Because the flap valve on the left atrial side normally overlaps the muscular rim to a greater or lesser extent, the PFO is a tunnel between the flap valve and the muscular rim. It is a channel for a right-to-left shunt when right atrial pressure exceeds that of the left, and it increases the risk for stroke. Owing to the adjacency of the PFO's left atrial opening to the anterior left atrial wall and the tendency of the tunnel to be narrow, it is seldom used as a portal for septal crossing without puncture. Furthermore, device closure of the PFO needs to take into account the antero-superior location of the opening and hence the proximity of the aortic root.

The septal pouch was described by Krishnan and Salazar as a new anatomic entity that potentially could be a site for thrombus formation. These investigators examined 94 autopsied hearts, focusing their attention on the pattern of fusion between the SP and SS. They found that 27% had a PFO; the remaining 68 hearts did not have a PFO. But they further observed that while 27 of these had complete closure along the entire surface of overlap between the SP and SS, in 41 there was incomplete fusion between the SP and SS, with a kangaroo-like pocket opening into the left atrium in 37 and into the right atrium in 4. The pouch opening was in the left atrium when the adhesion between the SS and SP was only at the margin of the SS (the inferior limit of the zone of overlap). When the adhesion was only at the free margin of the SP (the superior limit of overlap), the opening could be probed from the right atrium without entering the left atrium. They named the cleft resulting from this incomplete fusion the *septal pouch*, according to its appearance when filled with blood in the living. These authors hypothesized that the SP and SS come together at the time of birth and constant

movement against each other causes a friction-induced injury, leading to an inflammatory response that eventually results in fibrotic adhesion between the SP and SS. Moreover, this fusion starts at the caudal margin of the zone of overlap and continues in a cranial direction, explaining the more frequent location of a pouch opening in the left atrium when fusion is incomplete.

Whether the stagnant blood in this pocket (as in the left atrial appendage) may be a source of thrombus formation and cerebral and systemic embolic events is still unclear. Case reports have shown thrombus within the pouch and in the setting of cryptogenic stroke. Initial epidemiological studies are contradictory, both showing and not showing an association between the pouch and embolic cerebral events. In an editorial entitled *LA Septal Pouch as a Source of Thromboembolism: Innocent Until Proven Guilty?* Chandrashekhar and Narula synthesized the current uncertainty with the following sentence: "Before dismissing this entity into a footnote of medicine or before elevating it into a full member of the treatable stroke foci pantheon, we believe that this area still needs more robust evaluation. Future investigations will need to focus on…." Both CMR and CT provide cross-section slices that transect this region and may illustrate this particular anatomic feature, but we believe that 2D/3D TEE remains the best technique to image the septal pouch (Fig. 4.8).

As noted above, the FO and the interatrial groove constitute the extensive area that covers the medial wall of the left atrium. This area, with the exception of the septal pouch, is usually almost smooth. Rarely, however, a prominent ridge-like formation running laterally to the oval fossa extends to the atrial free wall (Fig. 4.9). Whether this ridge, which potentially may interfere with septal puncture or catheter navigation into the left atrium, is acquired or is due to a kind of "irregular" fusion between the SP and SS is unclear.

Figure 4.10 summarizes the different modalities of fusion between the septum primum and the infolding of atrial walls.

The Septal Atrio-ventricular Junction

The name *septal atrio-ventricular junction* refers to a specific area, the junction between the septal components of the atria and ventricles and the hingeline of the mitral and tricuspid leaflets. This region is centrally located in the heart and was named "crux cordis." Silverman and Schiller, in a paper entitled *Apex Echocardiography*, described this region with 2D TTE. By placing the transducer on the apex of the heart, they obtained a cross-sectional plane perpendicular to the septa and through the orifices of the atrio-ventricular valves, showing in a single image all four chambers of the heart. This section, now well-known as the *four-chamber view*, is one of the most informative echocardiographic

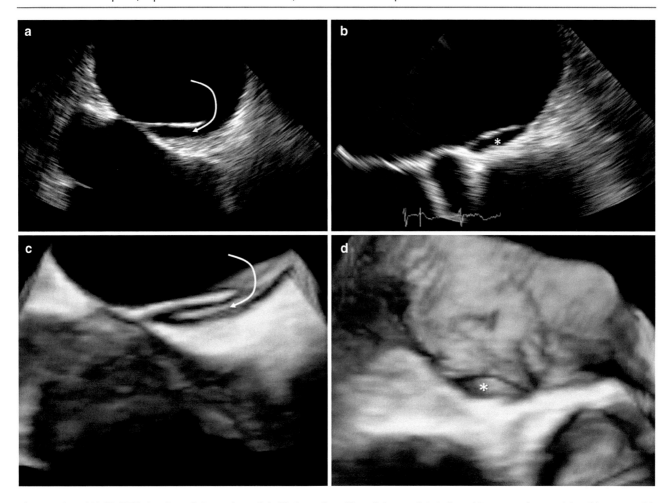

Fig. 4.8 (**a** and **b**) 2D TEE showing a left septal pouch in X plane; the orifice of the pouch is indicated by a curved arrow (**a**) and by an asterisk (**b**). (**c** and **d**) 3D TEE showing the equivalent cross sections

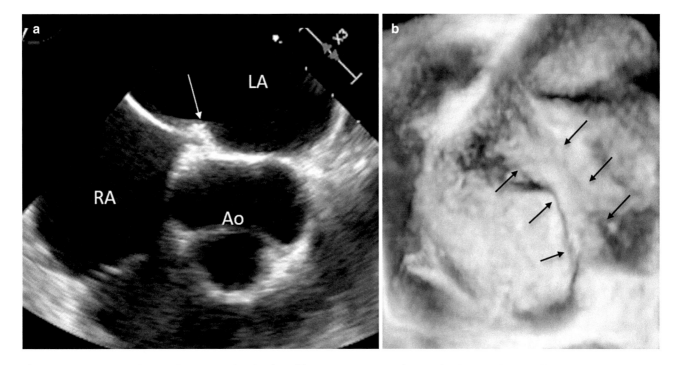

Fig. 4.9 2D (**a**) and 3D (**b**) TEE images showing the ridge-like structure (*arrows*) that may be due to an irregular fusion between the septum primum and the septum secundum

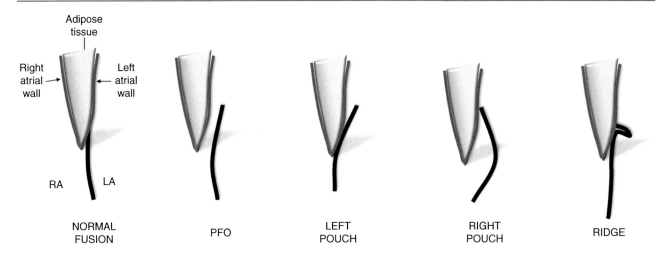

Fig. 4.10 Five modalities of fusion between the septum primum and the infolding of atrial walls (former septum secundum). The "irregular" fusion leading to a formation of a "ridge" is just an hypothesis. *PFO* patent foramen ovale

cross sections. The most peculiar anatomic feature of this area is the hingeline of the tricuspid septal leaflet, which is positioned more apically than the corresponding hinge of the mitral leaflet. The distance between the two hingelines in the normal adult heart should not exceed 8–9 mm/m². Because the tricuspid valve is always associated with the morphologic right ventricle, echocardiographers use this low insertion of the tricuspid septal leaflet to recognize the morphological right ventricle in complex congenital heart disease (*i.e.*, to correct transposition of great arteries).

Given this arrangement, the portion of the septum between the two hingelines is termed the *atrio-ventricular septum* (AVS) in that it separates the right atrium from the left ventricle. In the past, anatomists described the AVS as a muscular partition between the right atrium and left ventricle. More recently, new anatomic and histologic observations have shown that the AVS consists of the atrial wall on the right side and the crest of the interventricular septum on left side. Between these two muscular structures, there is a small amount of adipose tissue originating from the inferior pyramidal space (see below). For this particular anatomic arrangement, this area was re-named *atrioventricular muscular sandwich*, with the adipose tissue between the two muscular tissues representing the "meat" in the sandwich. Although the current noninvasive imaging techniques clearly can illustrate the atrio-ventricular region, they fail to distinguish this fine anatomical arrangement, which is beyond their spatial resolution power. In a few cases, when the adipose tissue is abundant enough to

separate the atrial wall from the ventricular crest, CMR is able to distinguish the adipose tissue between the muscular tissues (Fig. 4.11).

The adipose tissue located in the atrio-ventricular muscular sandwich is the anterior/superior continuation of the so-called inferior pyramidal space (IPS), which contains epicardial adipose tissue (Fig. 4.12). With the heart in anatomical orientation, the pyramid (or cone) has its base at the posterior/inferior surface of the heart; its superiorly located apex is at the central fibrous body. The IPS contains numerous important structures, including arteries, veins, and nerves. The most important arterial vessel is the atrioventricular nodal artery, which originates from the right coronary artery in 80% of individuals, and from the circumflex artery in the remaining 20%.

The Membranous Septum

Anteriorly, the hinge of the septal leaflet of the tricuspid valve divides the membranous septum (MS) into the atrioventricular membranous septum (AVMS), which separates the right atrium from the left ventricle, and the interventricular membranous septum (IVMS), which separates the left and the right ventricles. The superior margin of the MS is part of the fibrous tissue of the interleaflet triangle between the hingelines of the right-coronary and non-coronary aortic leaflets. Inferiorly, the MS inserts on the crest of the muscular interventricular septum (Fig. 4.13).

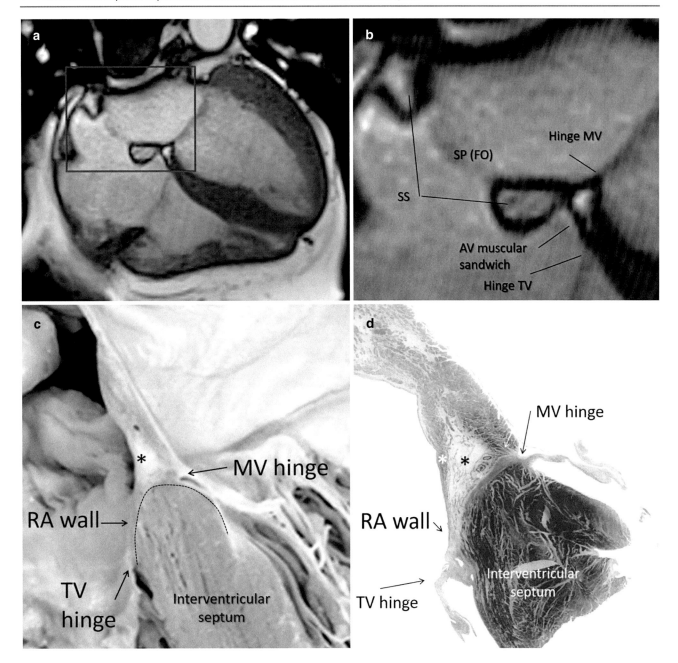

Fig. 4.11 (a) CMR cine sequence showing in a cross-sectional four-chamber view of the anatomic architecture of the septum primum (SP) at the fossa ovalis (FO) and the septum secundum (SS). (b) Magnified image of the red box in panel (a), showing the superior aspects of the septum secundum, near the atrial roof, and the inferior aspects, near the atrioventricular (AV) muscular sandwich. (c) Anatomic specimen showing the same structures. (d) Histologic section, with myocardium stained red and fibrous tissue stained green (Trichrome stain). *MV* mitral valve, *RA* right atrium, *TV* tricuspid valve, *black asterisk* indicates adipose tissue

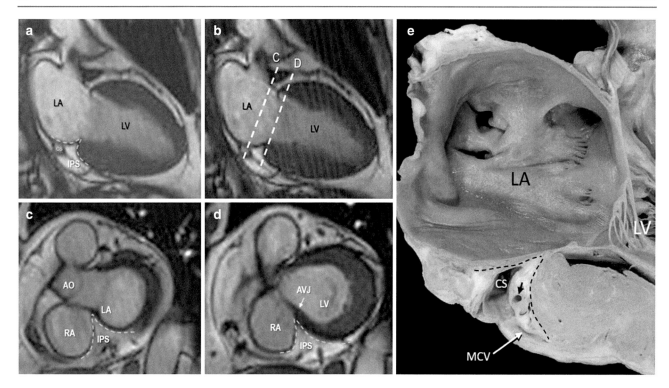

Fig. 4.12 CMR cine sequence still frames obtained with SSFP. (**a**) Two-chamber longitudinal plane showing the inferior pyramidal space (IPS) filled with epicardial adipose tissue (*yellow dotted line*) on the inferior-posterior aspect of the heart. (**b**) In the same image, the two dotted lines refer to the two short-axis planes shown in panels (**c**) and (**d**). (**c**) In this short-axis plane, the IPS is bordered by the walls of the right atrium (RA) and left atrium (LA). (**d**) In this lower short-axis

plane, the IPS is bordered by the right atrial wall and by the crest of the ventricular wall. (**e**) An anatomic specimen displayed in similar fashion as the image on panel (**a**). The IPS is located between the two *broken lines*. Within it are the coronary sinus (CS), the middle cardiac vein (MCV), and a coronary artery (*short arrow*). *Ao* aorta, *AVJ* atrioventricular junction, *LV* left ventricle

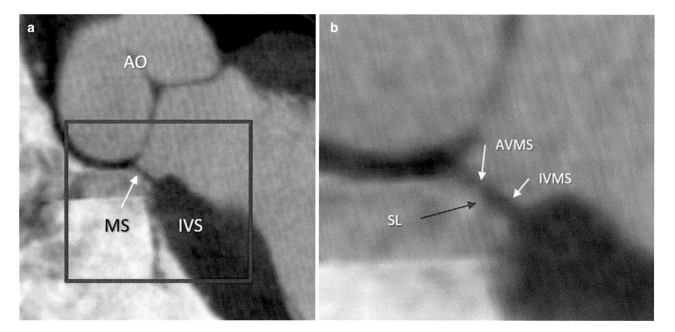

Fig. 4.13 CT scan (**a, b**) and 2D TEE (**c, d**) showing the membranous septum (MS) divided by the hingeline of the septal leaflet of the tricuspid valve (hinge) into the atrioventricular MS (AVMS) and the interven-

tricular MS (IVMS). Panels (**b**) and (**d**) are magnified images of the area inside the red box in panels (**a**) and (**c**)

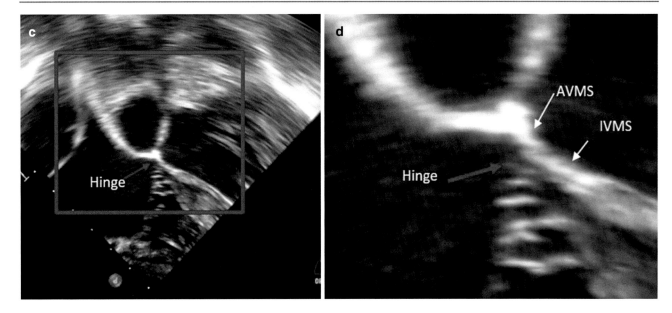

Fig. 4.13 (continued)

Suggested Reading

Anderson RH. Development of the atrial septum. Heart. 2016;102:481.

Anderson RH, Brown NA. The anatomy of the heart revisited. Anat Rec. 1996;246:1–7.

Anderson RH, Webb S, Brown NA. Clinical anatomy of the atrial septum with reference to its developmental components. Clin Anat. 1999;12:362–74.

Becker AE, Anderson RH. Atrioventricular septal defect. What's in a name? J Thorac Cardiovasc Surg. 1982;83:461–9.

Chandrashekhar Y, Narula J. LA septal pouch as a source of thromboembolism: Innocent until proven guilty? JACC Cardiovasc Imaging. 2010;3:1296–8.

Ferreira Martins JD, Anderson RH. Anatomy of the interatrial communications—What does the interventionist need to know? Cardiol Young. 2000;10:464–73.

Klimek-Piotrowska W, Hołda MK, Koziej M, Piątek K, Hołda J. Anatomy of the true interatrial septum for transseptal access to the left atrium. Ann Anat. 2016;205:60–4.

Krishnan SC, Salazar M. Septal pouch in the left atrium: a new anatomical entity with potential for embolic complications. JACC Cardiovasc Interv. 2010;3:98–104.

Ross J Jr, Braunwald E, Morrow AG. Transseptal left atrial puncture; new technique for the measurement of left atrial pressure in man. Am J Cardiol. 1959;3:653–5.

Silverman NH, Schiller NB. Apex echocardiography. A two-dimensional technique for evaluating congenital heart disease. Circulation. 1978;57:503–11.

Tugcu A, Okajima K, Jin Z, Rundek T, Homma S, Sacco RL, et al. Septal pouch in the left atrium and risk of ischemic stroke. JACC Cardiovasc Imaging. 2010;3:1276–83.

Wong JM, Lombardo DM, Barseghian A, Dhoot J, Hundal HS, Salcedo J, et al. Left atrial septal pouch in cryptogenic stroke. Front Neurol. 2015;6:57.

The Right Atrium and Left Atrium

5

Francesco F. Faletra, Laura A. Leo, Vera L. Paiocchi,
Susanne A. Schlossbauer, and Siew Yen Ho

The Right Atrium

This chapter describes the anatomy of the right and left atria using computed tomography (CT), cardiac magnetic resonance (CMR), and two-dimensional (2D) and three-dimensional (3D) transthoracic echocardiography (TTE) and transesophageal echocardiography (TEE), illustrated side-by-side with anatomic specimens where possible. Because these noninvasive techniques differ in their ability to visualize right atrial structures, this chapter begins by describing the advantages and limits of CT, CMR, and 2D/3D TTE and TEE.

Imaging Techniques

Computed Tomography

CT scans are certainly an excellent tool to visualize coronary arteries and left-side structures. The supremacy of CT over the other imaging techniques is due to the fact that the voxel (volume element) is a cube as small as 0.6 mm with the x, y, and z axis of equal dimensions (isotropic), allowing this technique to define boundaries of two adjacent structures that are as close as 0.6 mm to each other in all three spatial directions. Moreover, the system has the ability to observe a given organ, visualized in volume-rendering format, from different perspectives ("fly around") that allow an intuitive perception of the three-dimensionality.

Nevertheless, despite its superior spatial resolution, CT images of right-side structures are not of the same quality as those of the left-side counterparts. Routine CT scans are generally used to visualize left-side structures, and the acquisition modality follows a precise temporal protocol. Consequently, in routine practice the right atrial cavity is minimally opacified or not opacified at all. Achieving adequate and homogeneous opacification of the right atrium (RA) is difficult because of the mixing of nonopacified blood from the inferior vena cava (IVC) with the opacified blood from the superior vena cava (SVC). Moreover, streak and blooming artifacts resulting from contrast agent–opacified blood may reduce image quality and partially obscure RA structures. A specific protocol with a biphasic injection (the first injection with 100% contrast agent followed by a second injection with 50% contrast agent) may attenuate the streak artifacts and make the contrast in the RA more uniform. Other disadvantages of CT include exposure to ionizing radiation and risk for contrast agent–induced nephropathy. Moreover, obtaining images in motion with CT needs the acquisition of multiple phases (retrospective acquisition) with a relatively high radiation dose exposure (~10 mSv). The frame rate or temporal resolution (i.e., number of images per second) remains as low as 10–15 frames per second, making the motion appear less "naturally fluid" than with other imaging techniques. Despite these limitations, when the CT images are correctly acquired, the RA structure can be visualized beautifully. There are several post-processing imaging modalities for visualizing cardiac structures with CT. The most useful of these for visualizing RA structures are multiplanar reconstruction, which uses axial slices to create nonaxial 2D slices; volume-rendering images, an algorithm that transforms serially acquired axial slices into a volumetric data set; finally endocardial surface modality, an algorithm that makes the contrast transparent and thus allows visualization of the internal endocardial surface from any perspective.

F. F. Faletra (✉) · L. A. Leo · V. L. Paiocchi · S. A. Schlossbauer
Non-invasive Cardiovascular Imaging Department, Fondazione
Cardiocentro Ticino, Lugano, Switzerland
e-mail: Francesco.Faletra@cardiocentro.org;
lauraanna.leo@cardiocentro.org; vera.paiocchi@cardiocentro.org;
susanne.schlossbauer@cardiocentro.org

S. Y. Ho
Royal Brompton Hospital, Sydney Street, London, UK
e-mail: yen.ho@imperial.ac.uk

© Springer Nature Switzerland AG 2020
F. F. Faletra et al. (eds.), *Atlas of Non-Invasive Imaging in Cardiac Anatomy*, https://doi.org/10.1007/978-3-030-35506-7_5

Cardiac Magnetic Resonance (CMR)

As with CT, CMR is also intrinsically tridimensional, so it provides 3D volume-rendering for imaging of the external aspect of the heart. In clinical practice, CMR volume-rendering is used mainly to define the number, size, and positions of pulmonary veins (see below). CMR does not use radiation and provides "dynamic" images of the right chambers similar in quality to images of the left chambers. Theoretically, this imaging technique also should be able to reconstruct the internal structures of the RA in three dimensions, but in routine practice, CMR images are shown in 2D slices.

Echocardiography

The large difference in acoustic impedance between blood and cardiac structures allows echocardiography to visualize the internal surfaces of the heart with a high spatial and temporal resolution. However, because of the tomographic nature of both transthoracic (2D TTE) and transesophageal echocardiography (2D TEE), imaging of a given right atrial structure will be displayed only when the ultrasound beam directly transects the target structure. The best imaging ultrasound modality to visualize and "fly through" the internal surface of the RA is 3D transesophageal echocardiography (3D TEE). Indeed, the distance between the RA and the TEE transducer in the esophagus is "just right"—not so close as to have a narrow field of view and not so far as to lose image quality. Thus, by using 3D TEE, even small atrial structures are imaged with a richness of anatomical details secondary only to anatomic specimens. Unfortunately, the difference in acoustic impedance is not enough to distinguish between the external surface of the heart and surrounding structures. Thus, unless another medium (such as pericardial effusion) is in between, the external surfaces of the heart are substantially invisible to ultrasound.

Right Atrial Anatomy

The RA is located superior to the right ventricle and anterior and lateral to left atrium (LA). The RA receives venous blood from the two caval veins, from the coronary sinus, and from Thebesian veins, which are very minute channels that connect the right atrial cavity with medium-sized coronary veins. Anatomically, the RA can be divided in four main components: the *sinus venosus*, formed by the junction of the IVC and SVC and located posteriorly; the *right atrial appendage* (RAA), which is a large, triangular pouch extending laterally and anteriorly, partially covering the anterior aspect of the ascending aorta; the *vestibule*, which is the atrial outlet surrounding the tricuspid orifice; and the *interatrial septum*, also described as the medial wall of the RA. This last structure was extensively reviewed in Chap. 4.

Figure 5.1 illustrates a CT volume-rendering image of the external aspect of the RA from different perspectives (demonstrating "fly around"). The sinus node is located in the sulcus marking the cavo-atrial junction.

This chapter describes several right atrial structures that are particularly relevant for electrophysiologists: the terminal crest, the right atrial appendage (RAA), the cavo-tricuspid isthmus, and the Eustachian valve.

The Terminal Crest

The terminal crest (TC)—in Latin, *crista terminalis*—is a crescent-shaped muscular ridge on the endocardial surface that demarks the border between the smooth wall of the sinus venosus and the irregular wall of the RAA. The corresponding external aspect of the crest is called in Latin the *sulcus terminalis*. This groove is usually filled by epicardial adipose tissue (*see* Fig. 5.1). The TC varies from heart to heart in prominence, differing in thickness and width from a thin, almost invisible muscular line to a thick, broad-based muscular bump mimicking an atrial mass, but it is a constant anatomic feature of the RA. This muscular ridge originates in the proximity of the interatrial groove, runs laterally bordering the anterior aspect of the SVC orifice, and descends towards the IVC, where it splits into fine and finer muscular strands. An extensive array of pectinate muscles spreads perpendicularly or obliquely from the TC, lining the internal surface of the RAA, producing its "corrugated" surface. Although usually neglected by clinical cardiologists, the TC has been the subject of several detailed anatomic studies and electrophysiological investigations in recent decades. In fact, the TC has been shown to be a source of atrial tachycardias in patients without structural heart disease. Moreover, its muscular fiber architecture may act as a natural barrier to transverse conduction during typical atrial flutter. The TC has a clear conduction anisotropy, with a fast velocity of conduction in the longitudinal direction, corresponding to the predominantly longitudinal arrangement of its myocardial strands, and low velocity in its transverse direction, due to the lower density of side-to-side gap junctions.

Figure 5.2 shows the TC as visualized with CT multiplanar reconstruction and CT endocardial surface modality.

Figure 5.3 shows a large and protruding TC, a type easily mistaken for an atrial mass. The best view to visualize TC with 2D TEE is the bi-caval view, but 3D TEE offers superb images of the TC that mimic anatomic specimens. With its large field of view, 3D TEE enables the TC to be tracked along its entire curved course.

The Right Atrial Appendage

The RAA, derived from the embryological right atrium, has a broadly triangular shape and forms much of the anterior and lateral wall of the RA. It typically has an irregular internal surface due to the abundant pectinate muscles.

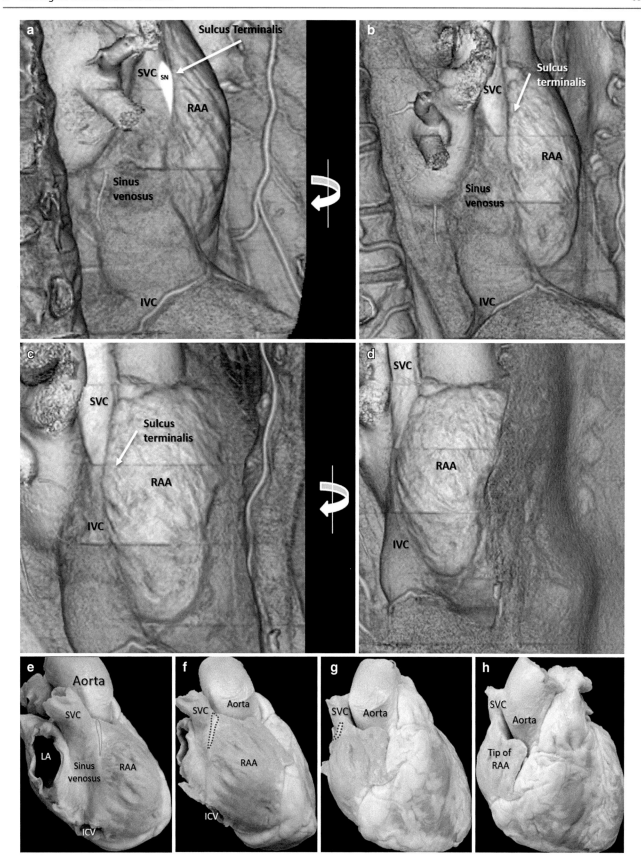

Fig. 5.1 (**a–d**) Volume-rendering CT scan showing in four different perspectives (fly around) the sinus venosus, the superior vena cava (SVC) and inferior vena cava (IVC), and the right atrial appendage (RAA). The sulcus terminalis divides the sinus venosus from the RAA. The white tadpole-shaped superimposed picture represents the sinus node (SN). (**e–h**) Different perspectives of the same heart viewed

from the right-posterior aspect (**e**) and rotated through to the anterior aspect (**h**). The sulcus terminalis filled with epicardial fat (*pale yellow*) is no longer a groove. The tip of the appendage points toward the aorta. The thin areas between the pectinate muscles are evident, appearing translucent. The red dotted areas mark the location of the sinus node

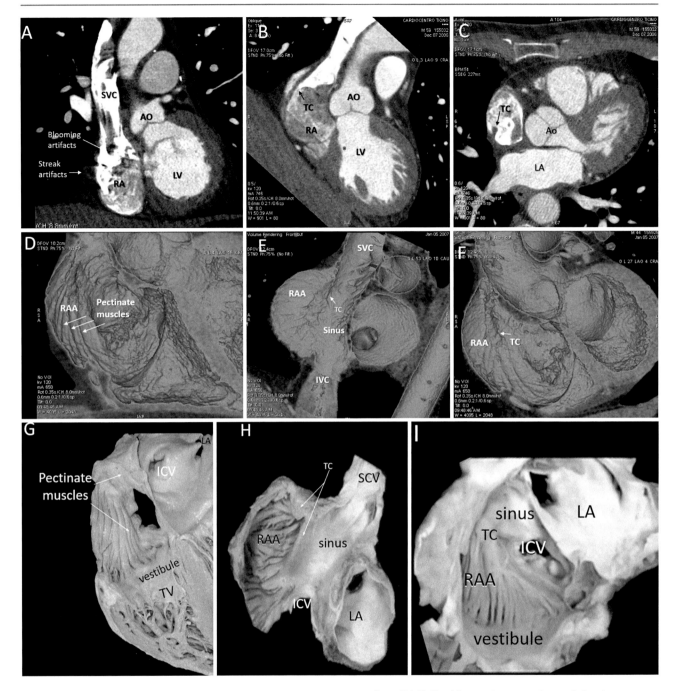

Fig. 5.2 The terminal crest (TC). (**a**) Multiplanar reconstruction showing the blooming and streak artifacts of the contrast flowing in the superior vena cava (SVC). (**b** and **c**) CT multiplanar slices showing the TC in a long-axis slice (**b**) and short-axis slice (**c**). (**d**–**f**) Endocardial surface modality showing from different perspectives the right atrial appendage (RAA) lined by pectinate muscles, and the sinus venosus (sinus). The *arrow* points at the TC. (**g**–**i**) Slices of heart specimens displaying the endocardial surface corresponding to images (**d**–**f**) respectively. Note the smooth-walled vestibule separating the pectinate muscles from the tricuspid valve (TV)

These protuberances are muscular bundles that arise almost perpendicularly from the TC, branching into finer bundles that connect irregularly with neighboring bundles to form a sort of a "dendritic" appearance between the TC and the smooth-walled vestibule. Thus, the atrial wall between the thicker pectinate muscles may be exceedingly thin, comprising only a few myocytes sandwiched between the epicardium and endocardium. The junction between the RAA and the RA is by far larger than the opening between the left atrial appendage (LAA) and the left atrium, allowing a more favorable "washing out" of blood flow. This characteristic may explain why in patients with atrial fibrillation the formation of thrombi is less common in the RAA than in the LAA. One of the pectinate muscles, known as the

Fig. 5.3 (**a**) Detail of 2D TTE four-chamber view showing a protrusion (*arrow*) in the right atrium (RA) due to a huge terminal crest (TC), often misdiagnosed as an atrial mass. (**b–d**) 2D TEE and 3D TEE bi-caval view in correct attitudinal orientation showing the TC between the orifice of the SVC and the RAA. (**e** and **f**) 3D TEE showing the entire curved course of the TC (*dotted line*) from two different oblique perspectives starting from the anterior aspect of the SVC orifice

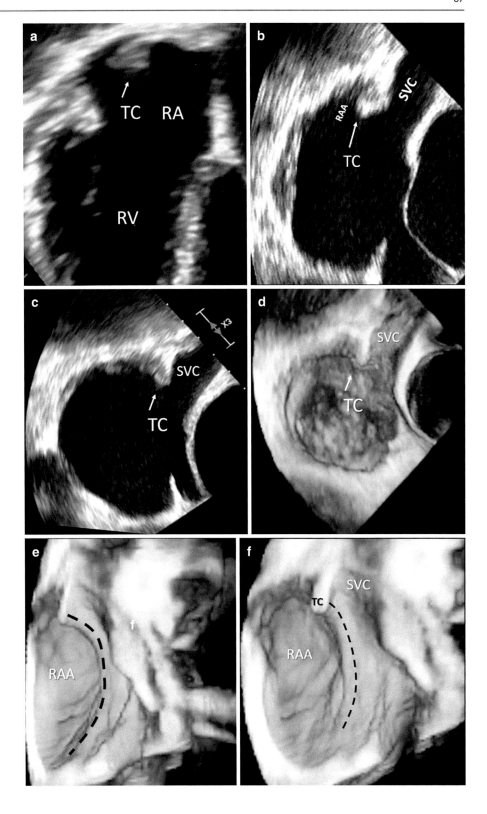

sagittal bundle (SB)—in Latin, the *tenia sagittalis* (sagittal worm)—is usually prominent and crosses the RAA wall transversely. It may form an incomplete ring around the tip portion of the RAA, delimiting an anterolateral pocket-shaped area of thin muscular wall. During lead implanta-

tion, the tip of the catheter could become stuck in this location. This pouch-like structure, indeed, provides a stable position for the lead and reduces the risk of dislodgement or stimulation of the phrenic nerve, but the electrophysiologist should be aware that the muscular wall between the pectinate muscles in this particular region is very thin and could be damaged by lead implantation. The external aspect of the RAA is best depicted by CT scans, whereas the internal surface is better seen by 2D and 3D TEE. 2D TEE has a better spatial resolution but depicts only a thin cross-sectional slice. 3D TEE provides a "panoramic" view of the internal surface of the RAA, showing the entire curved course of the SB (Fig. 5.4).

The Cavo-Tricuspid Isthmus

From an anatomical point of view, the cavo-tricuspid isthmus (CVTI) may be traced as almost a quadrilateral part of the inferior-posterior wall of the RA, delimited anteriorly by the tricuspid hinge line and posteriorly by the Eustachian valve. The medial and lateral borders are less distinct, corresponding to the coronary sinus ostium and to the final ramifications of the TC respectively (Fig. 5.5). The relevance of the CVTI for electrophysiologists is that it is the target of linear ablation to interrupt the macro-reentrant circuit of typical atrial flutter. CVTI ablation for typical atrial flutter is recognized to be the simplest, most straightforward, and best understood procedure, the one most likely to achieve complete success.

Indeed, electrophysiologists describe three isthmuses within the CVTI quadrilateral: para-septal, inferior, and inferolateral (Fig. 5.6). The preferred site of linear ablation is the inferior isthmus in the central sector, because the distance between the tricuspid valve hinge line and the orifice of the IVC is shorter in this sector than in the inferolateral isthmus, and it is further away from the atrioventricular node than the para-septal isthmus. Moreover, the wall of this sector is relatively thin and includes small areas of fatty-fibrous tissue that are electrically inert. These characteristics facilitate a completely transmural ablation line. However about 10% of patients have a sub-Eustachian pouch in the inferior isthmus, which may cause difficulties in achieving transmural lesions. In such cases, the longer inferolateral isthmus may be preferable.

Other anatomical variants such as prominent pectinate muscles, a tall and rigid Eustachian valve (EV), a long IVC-hinge line diameter, and angulation close to 90° between the IVC and CVTI may cause difficulties in catheter manipulation or in achieving optimal catheter-tissue contact. These issues may prolong the procedural time and increase the number of radiofrequency applications or result in gaps in the ablation line, which increase the risk of recurrence of the arrhythmias. Thus, *a priori* knowledge of the detailed anatomy of this region can significantly improve the safety and success rate of ablation procedures.

CT and CMR, performed before the onset of the procedure, are valid noninvasive imaging techniques for assessing these anatomical variants. CT also provides images of the variable course of the right coronary artery (RCA), which may be as close as 5 mm from the endocardial surface at the level of the inferolateral isthmus. CMR clearly shows the dynamicity of the CVTI, which shortens and lengthens during the cardiac cycle, but imaging of the EV or the hinge line of tricuspid leaflets is not always optimal. 3D TEE provides imaging of the entire surface of the CVTI in an *en face* view, allowing a precise definition of the para-septal, inferior, and inferolateral sectors, including the EV, coronary sinus ostium, tricuspid hinge line, and final ramifications of the TC. Moreover, rotation of the 3D data set allows 3D perspectives of the CVTI to be obtained that are similar to fluoroscopic left and right anterior oblique (LAO and RAO) projections. The technique may demonstrate those anatomic variants that may cause prolonged and difficult ablation procedures. Quantitative measurements are possible directly on 3D images. Because the echo machine is easily transportable into the electrophysiology lab, 3D TEE may guide ablation procedures. Recent data have shown that when used as a companion of fluoroscopy, 3D TEE significantly reduces the procedure time and radiation exposure. Thus, in selected patients in whom reducing fluoroscopic time is an important issue, the procedure may be guided by 3D TEE.

The Eustachian Valve

The Eustachian valve (EV) is a remnant of the embryonic right valve of the sinus venosus. It was first described by Eustachius in 1563. The function of the EV in fetal life is that of channeling umbilical oxygenated blood from the IVC across the patent foramen ovalis (PFO) to the systemic circulation. After birth, the EV does not appear to have any role, and in the adult population it almost disappears into a thin flap. In some individuals, however, a failure of reabsorption of the fetal EV may lead to a redundant, mobile membrane, and an incomplete and spot-like reabsorption produces a mesh of thin filaments (Chiari's network) (Fig. 5.7).

Both features may sometimes become a diagnostic puzzle. Usually both a large EV and Chiari's network are considered innocent echo findings. However, by maintaining a right atrial flow pattern toward the interatrial septum, they may favor persistence of a PFO or formation of an atrial septal aneurysm. Thrombosis or infective endocarditis on the EV has been reported sporadically in drug abusers. The Chiari network may have small thrombi attached to the filaments. When entangled with catheters entering the right atrium, small pieces of the network may break off and embolize. A large and prominent EV may be mistaken for a lower rim of an atrial septal defect or may complicate a percutaneous PFO closure. Finally, a prominent and thick EV may make for catheter manipulation more difficult during CVTI ablation.

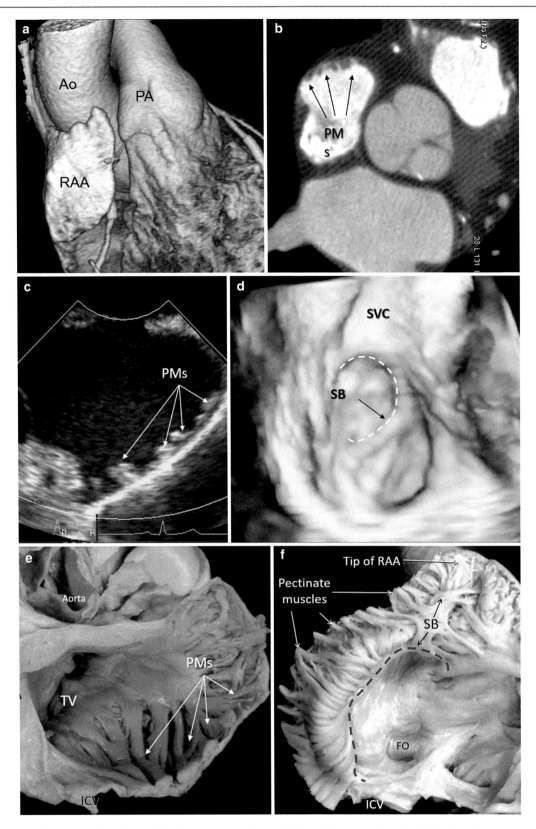

Fig. 5.4 Right atrial appendage (RAA). (**a**) CT volume-rendering format shows the external aspect of the RAA. This format shows that the RAA has a triangle-shaped configuration and extends laterally and anteriorly, partially wrapping the aortic root (Ao). (**b**) CT multiplanar reconstruction shows in cross-sectional format the array of pectinate muscles (PM). (**c**) Magnified image of 2D TEE showing a cross-sectional slice of the RAA. (**d**) Magnified 3D TEE image showing the *en face* view of the of the RAA. 2D and 3D TEE show pectinate muscles (PMs) and the sagittal bundle (SB), which forms an incomplete ring (*white dotted line*). (**e**) The posterior parts of the RA have been removed from this specimen to provide a view of the pectinate muscles and thin walls (*small arrows*) in a display similar to image (**c**). (**f**) The wall of the RAA has been deflected posteriorly, revealing the fossa ovalis (FO) enface. The *blue broken line* marks the course of the TC. The SB arises from the superior course of the TC

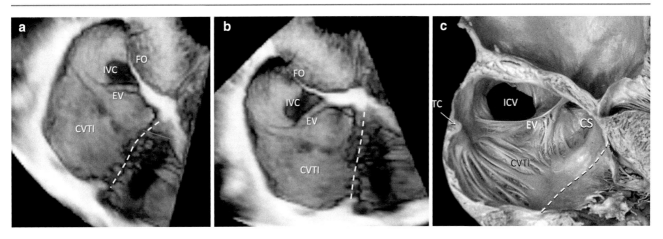

Fig. 5.5 (a and b) Two different 3D TEE perspectives showing the cavo-tricuspid isthmus (CVTI), the Eustachian valve (EV), the inferior vena cava (IVC), and the fossa ovalis (FO). The dotted lines mark the hinge line of the tricuspid valve. (c) A heart specimen displayed in similar fashion. *CS* coronary sinus, *TC* terminal crest

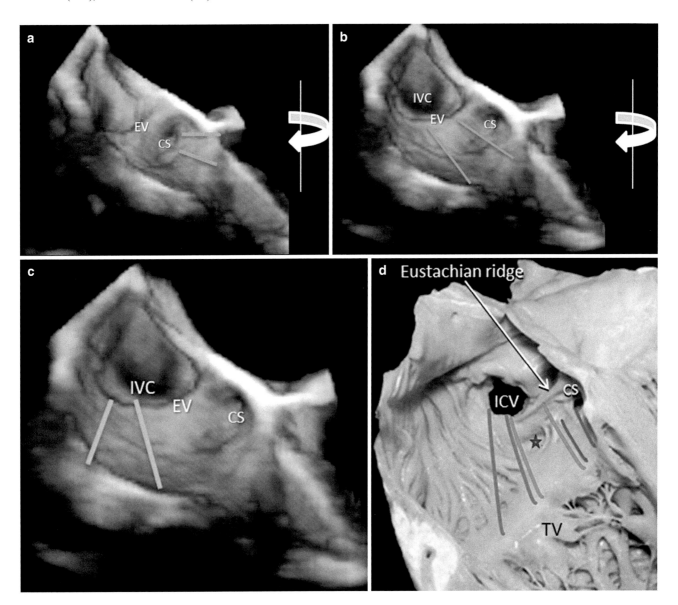

Fig. 5.6 (a) This 3D TEE image shows the para-septal sector (*two orange lines*) of the CVTI. (b) A right-to-left rotation around the y axis reveals the inferior sector (*two blue lines*). (c) Further rotation shows the inferolateral sector (*two green lines*). (d) The three CVTI sectors marked correspondingly on an image of a heart specimen. Note the depression of a pouch (*star*) in the inferior sector. The Eustachian valve is rudimentary in this heart, but the Eustachian ridge is moderately prominent

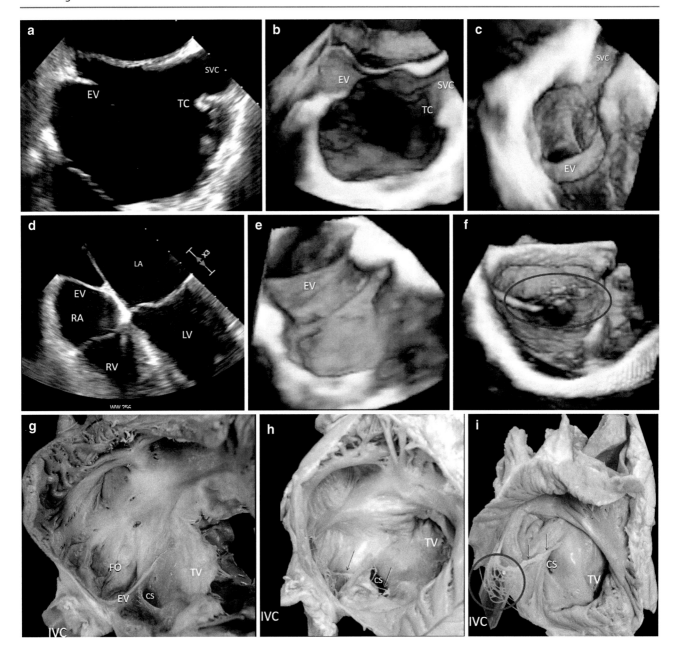

Fig. 5.7 (**a**) 2D TEE bi-caval view showing a normal-sized Eustachian valve (EV). (**b**) Similar image in 3D perspective. (**c**) EV seen in *en face* view. (**d**) 2D TEE four-chamber view showing a very large EV. (**e**) 3D TEE showing a large EV in *en face* view. (**f**) Chiari's network (*red ellipse*). (**g** and **h**) Dissected right atria displayed in simulated right-anterior oblique (RAO) view. (**g**) shows a typical EV; in (**h**) the EV is a Chiari network (*arrows*) that also involves the Thebesian valve at the coronary sinus (CS). (**i**) The Chiari network (*arrows*) is displayed by putting a tube into the orifice of the inferior vena cava (IVC) (*red circle*). *LA* left atrium, *LV* left ventricle, *RA* right atrium, *RV* right ventricle, *SVC* superior vena cava, *TC* terminal crest, *TV* tricuspid valve

The Left Atrium

The left atrium (LA) is an ovoid-shaped chamber that receives pulmonary venous blood through the pulmonary veins that enter the back of the chamber. It is the most posterior chamber of the heart, located adjacent to the esophagus and descending thoracic aorta, and is slightly superior and to the left of the right atrium. Anteriorly, the LA lies just behind the transverse sinus and the aortic root. Inferiorly, this cham-ber is bordered by the vestibule, the LA outlet surrounding the mitral valve orifice. Superiorly, the "roof" of the LA receives the entrance of the superior pulmonary veins, and the right pulmonary artery passes above it. The anteromedial wall comprises the interatrial septum, and the lateral wall includes the left atrial isthmus (LAI) and a small, finger-like left atrial appendage (LAA). The internal surface of the LA is rather smooth, except for the presence of pectinate muscles in the LAA (Fig. 5.8).

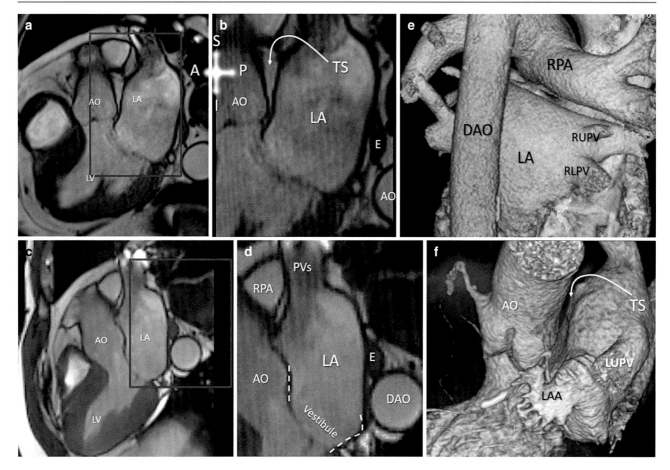

Fig. 5.8 (**a–d**) Cardiac MR images showing the anatomical relationship between the left atrium (LA) and surrounding structures. The areas in the red box of (**a**) and (**c**) are magnified in (**b**) and (**d**) respectively. Anteriorly, the LA lies posterior to the transverse sinus (TS) and aorta (AO). Posteriorly, the LA is adjacent to the esophagus (E) and descending thoracic aorta (DAO). Superiorly, the LA borders the right pulmonary artery (RPA) and receives the entrance of the pulmonary veins (PVs). Inferiorly, the LA ends with the vestibule (*dotted lines*). (**e**) CT volume-rendering image showing the posterior aspect of the LA and the spatial relationship with the DAO and RPA. (**f**) CT volume-rendering image showing the lateral aspect of the LA and the left atrial appendage (LAA) and the spatial relationship with the ascending aorta (AO) and TS

Physiology of the Left Atrium

Some insights on the physiology of the LA will be useful because of its clinical impact. The LA modulates left ventricular filling and cardiac performance through its roles as a reservoir, conduit, and booster pump (Fig. 5.9).

The *reservoir phase* stores the pulmonary venous flow in the LA cavity during left ventricular (LV) systole and isovolumetric relaxation. In this phase, the LA reaches its maximal volume. This phase depends on atrial compliance and LV longitudinal systolic shortening. Because the apex of the heart is firmly fixed at the diaphragm, the longitudinal systolic LV shortening determines an increase in the LA cavity, through the descent of the mitral annulus plane. The increase of LA volume leads to a diminution in the LA pressure and, by creating an intracavitary "suction effect," develops a pressure gradient between the pulmonary veins (PVs) and the LA, which facilitates PV inflow into the LA. Thus, the LA reservoir function is greatly influenced by the LV longitudinal systolic shortening. The LV systolic shortening is therefore a sensitive index of LV performance. This index may be reduced not only in clinically manifest dilated and hypertrophic cardiomyopathies (where this longitudinal shortening is greatly reduced or even abolished) but also in the first stages of ischemic heart disease. When this happen, the LA volume does not increase, causing a rise of LA pressure and a reduction of the PVs–LA pressure gradient. Stasis in PVs and pulmonary capillaries eventually results in the classic symptoms of heart failure. Because the radial LV contraction is preserved, as the ejection fraction, this clinical condition is now referred to as *heart failure with preserved ejection fraction*.

In the *conduit phase*, the LA transfers blood passively into the LV during diastole. This phase can be divided into two parts: the early phase and the diastasis phase.

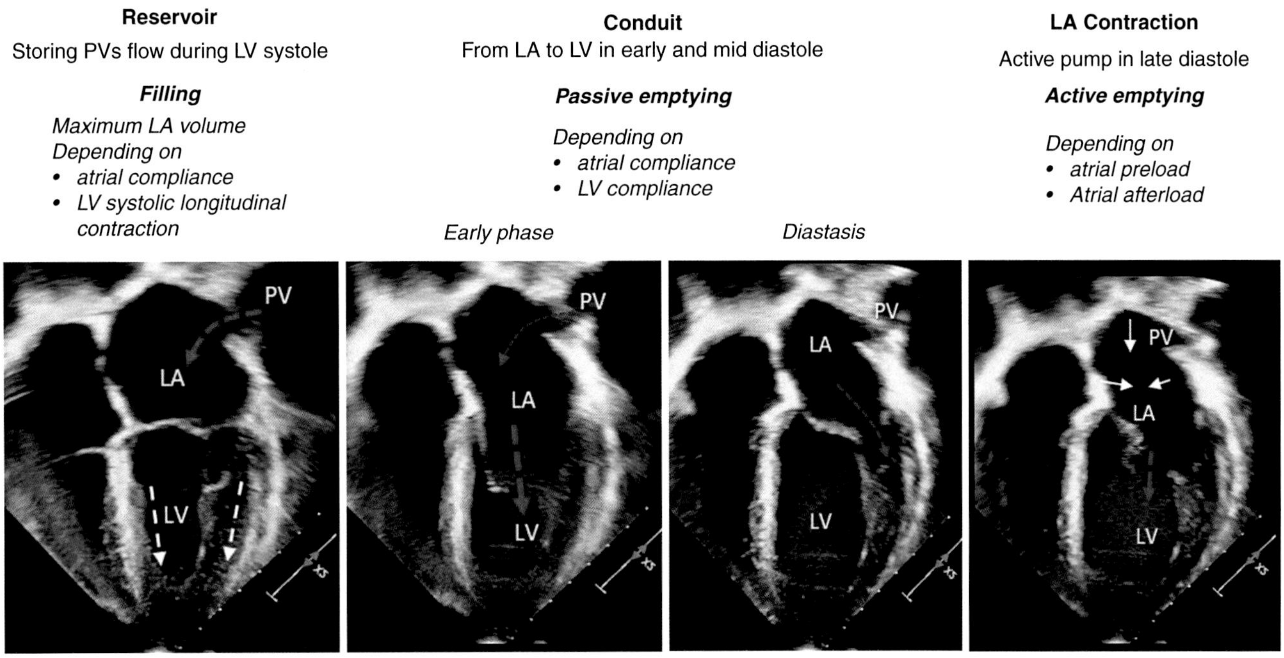

Reservoir	Conduit	LA Contraction
Storing PVs flow during LV systole	From LA to LV in early and mid diastole	Active pump in late diastole
Filling	*Passive emptying*	*Active emptying*
Maximum LA volume *Depending on* • *atrial compliance* • *LV systolic longitudinal* *contraction*	*Depending on* • *atrial compliance* • *LV compliance* *Early phase* *Diastasis*	*Depending on* • *atrial preload* • *Atrial afterload*

Fig. 5.9 The phases of LA function illustrated by 2D transthoracic echocardiography. The white dotted lines represent the systolic longitudinal shortening of the left ventricle (LV). The red dotted lines represent the flow. *LA* left atrium, *PV* pulmonary vein

Both phases depend on LA and LV compliance. In the early phase, the pressure of the LA overcomes the pressure of the LV, the mitral valve opens, and a "torrential" flow enters the LV. In the diastasis phase, LA pressure equals LV pressure, and for an instant the heart is completely still. These two parts of the conduit phase correspond to the A wave and plateau of pulsed wave (PW) Doppler and M-mode echocardiography.

The *atrial contraction* works as an efficient booster pump. It reflects the force of atrial contractility and is influenced by the atrial preload (i.e., the amount of venous return) and atrial afterload (i.e., LV end-diastolic pressures). To maintain cardiac output, the atrial booster pump function is increased with age, owing to the physiological reduction of LV compliance. The booster pump function is lost in atrial fibrillation. This loss is associated with a fall in cardiac output. The atrial contraction corresponds to the E wave of PW Doppler and M-mode echocardiography.

Structures of the Left Atrium

This section describes several pertinent structures of the LA: the left atrial isthmus (LAI), the LAA, the left lateral ridge (LLR), and the pulmonary veins (PVs).

The Left Atrial Isthmus

The LAI comprises of the inferior-lateral wall of the LA between the left lower pulmonary vein (LLPV) and the mitral annulus. This area has no specific boundaries or landmarks and is generally smooth, except for irregularities such as small pits and crevices around the orifice of the LAA. Interestingly, although the LAI is almost disregarded by general cardiologists, it is a relevant target for electrophysiologists. A linear ablation lesion connecting the medial border of the LLPV orifice up to the lateral commissure of the mitral annulus may interrupt a flutter circuit around the mitral annulus or may terminate an atrial fibrillation resistant to isolation of PVs (Fig. 5.10). A potential complication of ablating in this area is damage to the left circumflex artery or coronary sinus, both of which run in close proximity to the epicardial aspect of the LAI.

Left Atrial Appendage

The LAA is a remnant of the fetal left atrium, which forms during the fourth week of embryonic development. It appears as a small, finger-like protrusion originating from the smooth left atrial cavity.

Physiology of the LAA

The LAA has physiological characteristics distinct from the rest of the atrial cavity, which are sometimes controversial. In the past, the LAA was considered to be a relatively insignificant portion of cardiac anatomy; some authors described it as "the most useless and lethal appendix of our body," referring to the fact that thrombi have the predilection to form within the LAA in patients with

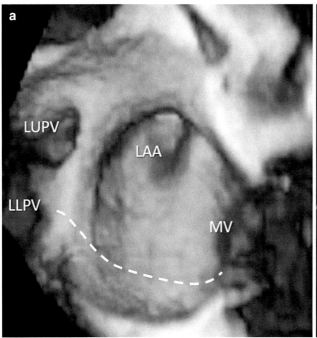
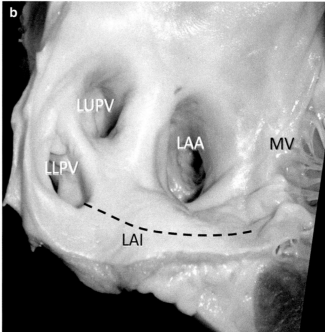

Fig. 5.10 (**a**) 3D TEE image of the left atrial isthmus (LAI) seen from an oblique perspective. The dotted line is where electrophysiologists perform a linear ablation between the left lower pulmonary vein

(LLPV) and the hingeline of the mitral valve (MV). (**b**) Anatomical specimen in a similar orientation. *LAA* left atrial appendage, *LUPV* left upper pulmonary vein

atrial fibrillation. The concept that the LAA is merely a remnant of the fetal left atrium that has no function in adult life, only playing a role in causing disease (thromboembolism), is incorrect. In fact, several beneficial functions can be attributed to the LAA in normal individuals:

- The LAA has greater compliance than the remaining "smooth" left atrium, and its ability to act as reserve of blood volume has been demonstrated by the fact that the compliance of the entire atrial cavity is reduced when the LAA is removed. Moreover, in humans, a temporary clamping of the LAA during cardiac surgery results in an increase in left atrial pressure and dimensions and in trans-mitral and pulmonary diastolic flow velocities.
- The LAA contributes to the systolic stroke volume; its contraction, in fact, adds a further quota of blood to ventricular filling.
- The LAA is an endocrine organ. Its myocytes have a concentration of atrial natriuretic factor (ANF) 40 times greater than those of any other heart cavity. It appears, therefore, to be a highly sensitive organ in the regulation of cardiac volume: lengthening of its muscular fibers (as occurs in overload volume) causes an increase in release of ANF that promotes diuresis and vasodilation, and vice versa.
- Finally, there is some evidence that the LAA plays a role in regulating thirst in hypovolemia.

Anatomy of the LAA

Externally, the LAA lies anterolaterally, covering the atrioventricular groove, in close proximity to the left circumflex artery. Characteristically, the LAA shows a narrow neck where it joins with the atrial chamber but has variability in terms of volume, shape, and size. Externally, its morphology may be classified into four types: "chicken wing," "cauliflower," "cactus," and "windsock." The chicken-wing morphology signifies an angulation within the body of the appendage. The cauliflower morphology has many small lobes with a complex architecture, without a dominant lobe. The cactus morphology has a dominant central lobe and several secondary lobes. In practice, however, the cauliflower and cactus morphologies may be indistinguishable, as both are short and stumpy. Finally, the windsock morphology represents a single dominant central lobe without a significant bend. This classification is far from clear-cut when examining the LAA in heart specimens or on preparations of casts made from the insides of the LAA (Fig. 5.11). The same cast can sometimes show two different shapes depending on the perspective from which it is viewed; it may be more practical to consider two main types: short or long, with or without a bend.

The internal aspect is even more complex, with numerous pectinate muscles delimiting lobes of different sizes and shapes. A narrow orifice joins the LAA with the smooth venous component of the left atrium. This anatomic configuration favors blood stasis and thrombi formation, especially in the absence of vigorous LAA contraction, as in case of atrial fibrillation (Fig. 5.12).

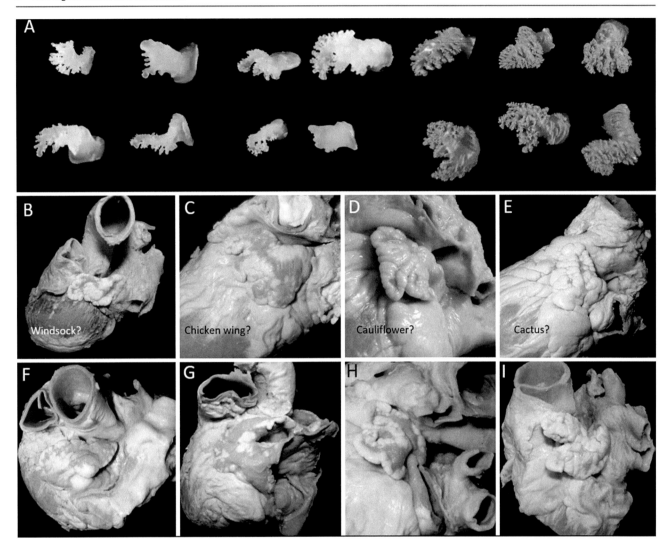

Fig. 5.11 (a) Endocasts of the left atrial appendage (LAA) from 14 adult heart specimens, showing some of the variety of shapes and sizes. (b–e) The external appearance of the LAA as viewed from the side of the heart is shown with variable coverage of epicardial fat that obscures the lobes used to classify the LAA shapes. Examples of unusual variants include (f) tip and half LAA folded over; (g) sharp bend with tip lodged in the transverse sinus; (h) short and bifid; (i) two long appendages with a common opening into the LA

Recognizing these different morphologies may be helpful in planning the type and size of LAA closure devices for percutaneous catheter implantation. This procedure is now considered a reasonable alternative to reduce the risk of cerebrovascular events in patients with atrial fibrillation for whom anticoagulation is contraindicated. Thus, a detailed quantitative anatomy of the LAA for patients undergoing LAA closure is "condition sine qua non" for the selection of the device size that best matches LAA size and shape. Both CT and TEE provide diagnostic images of the LAA on which quantitative parameters can be measured.

Imaging of the LAA
Because of its high spatial resolution, CT should be considered the ideal imaging technique for visualizing the LAA. The volume-rendering format shows its position, shape, and spatial relationship with surrounding structures. The multiplanar reconstruction allows a precise quantitative assessment of the size of the orifice and the length of the body (Fig. 5.13).

For its versatility and its high temporal and spatial resolution, multiplanar 2D TEE remains the primary imaging modality for imaging the LAA; it is the gold standard for ruling out thrombi (Fig. 5.14a–c). Because the LAA is relatively close to the esophagus and is relatively small, it is an ideal structure to be visualized by 3D TEE. Indeed, the entire LAA can be included in a narrow 3D TEE data set, which allows a high spatial and temporal resolution producing images of exquisite quality. Moreover, with this imaging technique, the orifice can be seen in *en face* perspective (Fig. 5.14d–f); longitudinal cuts reveal its cross-sectional aspects with the distribution of lobes and pectinate muscles (Fig. 5.14g–i).

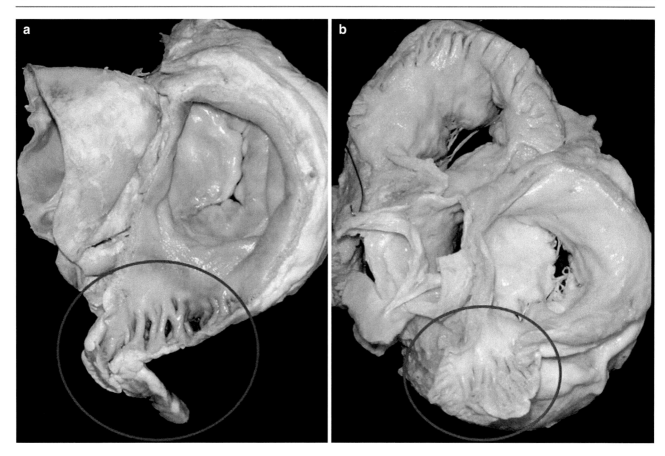

Fig. 5.12 (**a** and **b**) Anatomic specimens showing the variable arrangement of the internal aspect of the LAA (*red circles*)

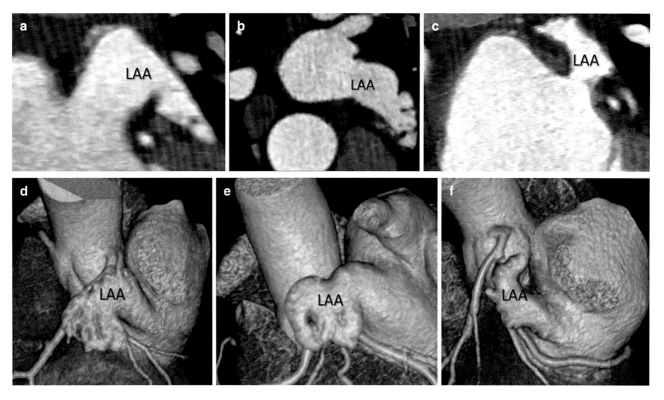

Fig. 5.13 CT multiplanar reconstruction (**a–c**) and volume-rendering format (**d–f**) showing the extremes in the shape of the LAA

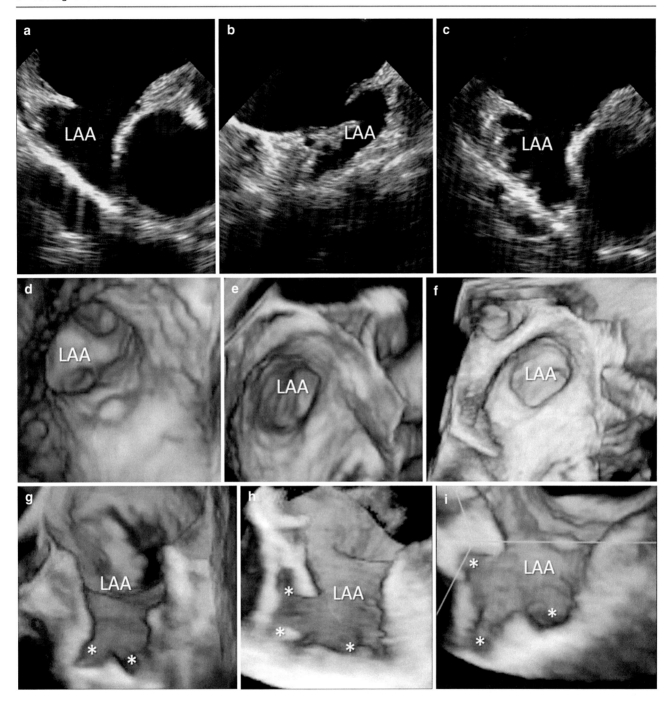

Fig. 5.14 (**a–c**) 2D TEE showing the different cross-sectional aspects of the LAA. (**d–f**) 3D TEE *en face* views showing the variable size of the LAA orifice. (**g–i**) 3D TEE cross-sections showing the distribution of the lobes (*asterisks*)

The Left Lateral Ridge

A muscular ridge can be found between the orifices of the pulmonary veins (PVs) and the LAA. This ridge is the most prominent structure of the LA and is described by anatomists as the left lateral ridge (LLR) (Fig. 5.15). Over the decades, however, this structure has been named differently. Because it may have a bulbous tip, it was frequently mistaken for a thrombus or mass protruding into the LA at the time of the initial 2D TEE examinations. For this reason, it is also known as the "coumadin ridge." In reality, the LLR is an infolding of the lateral atrial wall slightly protruding into the left atrial cavity. Nerve bundles, adipose tissue, small atrial arteries, and the remnant of the vein of Marshall (or its ligament) are sited within the fold. This vein (also known as the oblique left atrial vein) joins the great cardiac vein at the point where the latter becomes the coronary sinus. It is the remnant of the

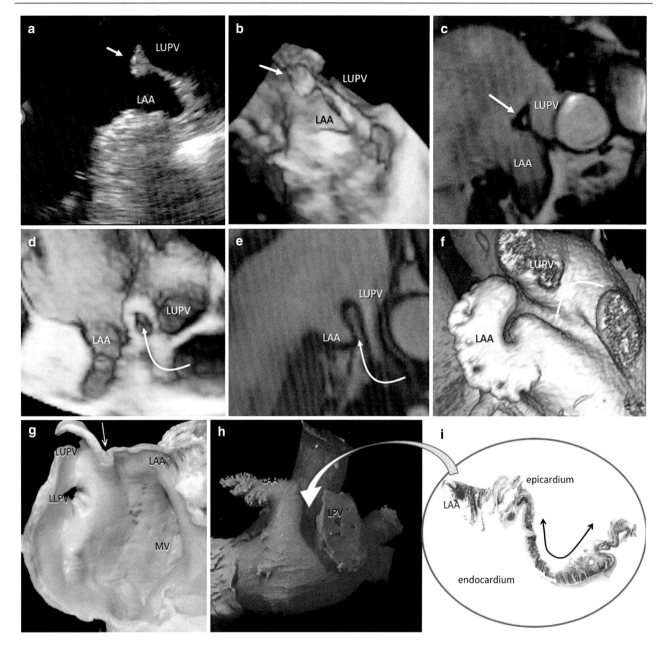

Fig. 5.15 The left lateral ridge (LLR) may have a bulbous tip (*arrow*), as seen on 2D TEE (**a**), 3D TEE (**b**), and CMR (**c**). At the beginning of 2D TEE examinations, it was frequently mistaken for a thrombus or mass protruding in the LA. The LLR is an infolding of the atrial wall (*curved arrow*), as seen on 3D TEE (**d**), CMR (**e**), and volume-rendering CT (**f**). An anatomical specimen (**g**), an endocast (**h**), and a histological image (**i**) show the infolding architecture of the LLR

embryonic left superior cardinal vein; when patent along its entire length, this is persistence of the left superior caval vein. Normally obliterated, this venous structure is patent in some patients for a centimeter or more from its juncture with the great cardiac vein/coronary sinus. Myocardial fibers and nerves adjacent to the vein of Marshall have been implicated as a source of ectopic beats, initiating paroxysmal tachyarrhythmias or atrial fibrillation. Thus, the vein of Marshall,

along with PVs, has been targeted for ablation. Because of the presence of this vein, electrophysiologists may call the LLR the "ligament of Marshall."

On the endocardial surface, the width of this ridge is not uniform (ranging from 3 to 6 mm), and it presents a varied profile in an anatomic study: rounded (75%), flat top (15%), and pointed (10%). Because it is part of the muscular wall of the left atrium, the LLR has its own contractility, becoming

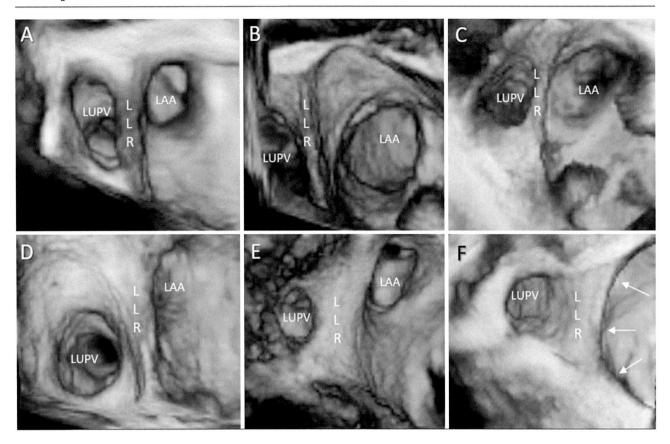

Fig. 5.16 (**a–e**) 3D TEE from an overhead perspective, showing different shapes of the LLR, along with the left atrial appendage (LAA) and left upper pulmonary vein (LUPV). (**f**) 3D TEE from an overhead/oblique perspective showing that the LLR has a convex profile (*arrows*)

thicker and more convex during atrial systole. The variable size and shape of the ridge may create difficulties in catheter contact and stability when ablating the orifices of the left PVs (Fig. 5.16).

Pulmonary Veins

The PVs join the left atrium by entering the posterior-superior part of the cavity. About 70% of the population has two veins from each lung. The pulmonary flow from the right superior and middle lobes is collected by the right upper pulmonary vein (RUPV). The left upper pulmonary vein (LUPV) drains the left superior lobe and the lingula, while the right lower pulmonary vein (RLPV) and left lower pulmonary vein (LLPV) drain the corresponding inferior lobes (Fig. 5.17).

Anatomical variants are frequent. In about 15% of the population, the left upper and lower PVs merge into a common trunk; on the right side, an accessory vein entering independently is rather common (Fig. 5.18).

The PV orifices are oval rather than round. The intervenous ridge, is the region between two separate ipsilateral veins. Usually PVs enter gradually into the atrial cavity, assuming a funnel-shaped configuration that makes the precise site of the venous-atrial junction difficult to identify. Histologically, the distal part of the veins (near their entry into the atrial cavity) is covered by an extension of the electrically active layer of atrial myocardium, with a discontinuous pattern of distribution along the vessels. This irregular pattern may cause abnormal electrical activity (i.e., ectopic beats, local re-entry, sustained focal activity), which may eventually trigger an atrial fibrillation. Indeed, the most common interventional treatment for symptomatic drug-resistant atrial fibrillation is the electrical isolation of PVs. A pre-procedural CT or CMR definition of the number, size, and shape of PVs is therefore relevant for an effective procedure and for follow-up in case of PV stenosis.

The volume-rendering modality of CT provides a precise anatomical picture of the four PVs, but images of individual orifices of the PVs can be seen *en face* with surprising clarity and spatial resolution using 3D TEE. On the other hand, CMR is uniquely able to detect myocardial fibrosis (scar tissue). Using late gadolinium enhancement (LGE), regions with fibrosis exhibit high signal intensity. Usually LGE is used to reveal fibrosis in ventricular myocardium, but it may

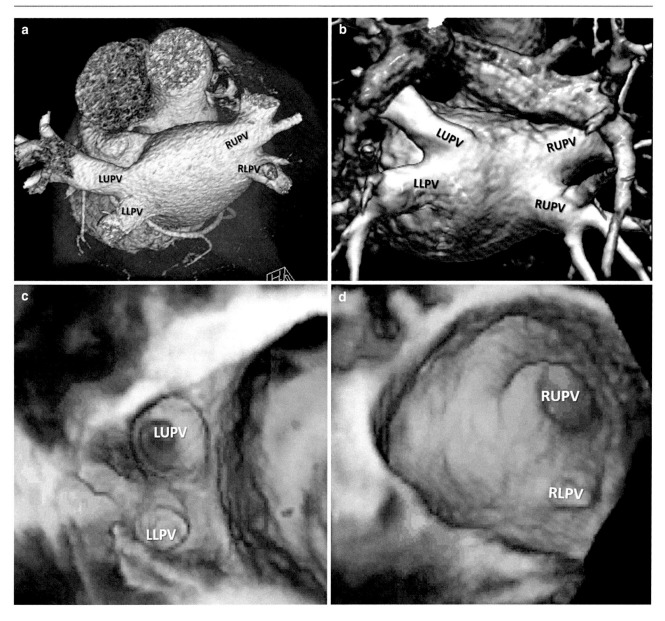

Fig. 5.17 The four pulmonary veins, as shown by the CT volume-rendering modality (**a**) and CMR 3D angiographic volume-rendering (**b**). 3D TEE (**c**) showing the internal orifices of the left upper pulmo-nary vein (LUPV) and left lower pulmonary vein (LLPV). 3D TEE (**d**) showing the internal orifices of the right upper pulmonary vein (RUPV) and the right lower pulmonary vein (RLPV)

also be adapted to detect atrial or PV fibrosis. It may be speculated that extension of post-ablation fibrosis around PVs is correlated with effectiveness of the ablation. Nevertheless, CT remains the most informative imaging technique: along with the anatomy of the PVs, it can reveal the status of coronary arteries, the absence of thrombi inside the LAA, and precise measurements of the LAA orifice and depth.

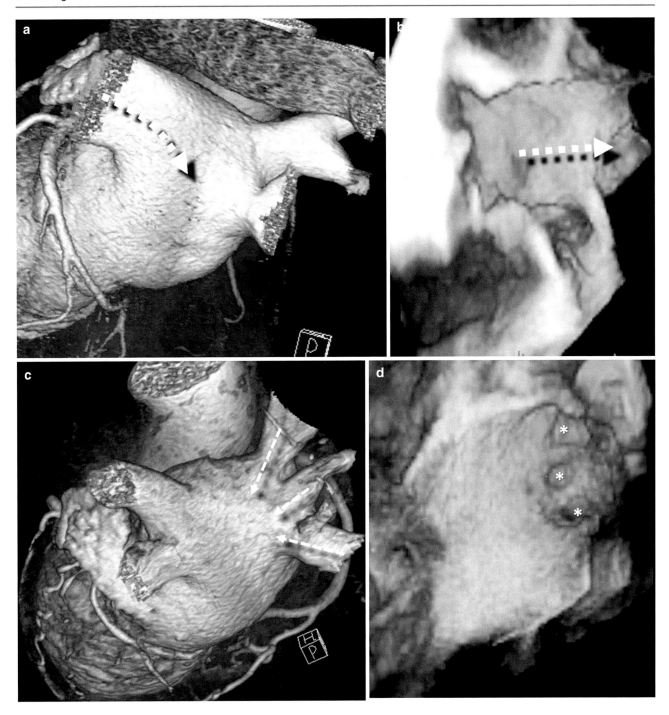

Fig. 5.18 (**a**) CT volume-rendering scan of a patient with a left common trunk (*dotted arrow*). (**b**) Longitudinal cross-sectional 3D TEE image showing a common trunk (*dotted arrow*). (**c**) CT volume-rendering scan of a patient with an accessory right pulmonary vein entering independently into the LA (*dotted arrows*). (**d**) 3D TEE showing the orifices (*asterisks*) of three right pulmonary veins

Suggested Reading

Anderson RH, Ho SY, Brecker SJ. Anatomy: anatomic basis of cross-sectional echocardiography. Heart. 2001;85:716–20.

Becker AE. Left atrial isthmus: anatomic aspects relevant for linear catheter ablation procedures in humans. J Cardiovasc Electrophysiol. 2004;15:809–12.

Cabrera JA, Sanchez-Quintana D, Ho SY, Medina A, Anderson RH. The architecture of the atrial musculature between the orifice of the inferior caval vein and the tricuspid valve: the anatomy of the isthmus. J Cardiovasc Electrophysiol. 1998;9:1186–95.

Faletra FF, Ho SY, Auricchio A. Anatomy of right atrial structures by real-time 3D transesophageal echocardiography. JACC Cardiovasc Imaging. 2010;3:966–75.

Ho SY. Pulmonary vein ablation in atrial fibrillation: does anatomy matter? J Cardiovasc Electrophysiol. 2003;14:156–7.

Ho SY, McCarthy KP, Faletra FF. Anatomy of the left atrium for interventional echocardiography. Eur J Echocardiogr. 2011;12:i11–5.

Kalman JM, Olgin JE, Karch MR, Hamdan M, Lee RJ, Lesh MD. "Cristal tachycardias": origin of right atrial tachycardias from the crista terminalis identified by intracardiac echocardiography. J Am Coll Cardiol. 1998;31:451–9.

Loukas M, Tubbs RS, Tongson JM, Polepalli S, Curry B, Jordan R, Wagner T. The clinical anatomy of the crista terminalis, pectinate muscles and teniae sagittalis. Ann Anat. 2008;190:81–7.

The Left and Right Ventricles

6

Francesco F. Faletra, Laura A. Leo, Vera L. Paiocchi,
Susanne A. Schlossbauer, Giovanni Pedrazzini,
Tiziano Moccetti, and Siew Yen Ho

As in the previous chapters, the three imaging techniques will be used to illustrate anatomy. In this chapter we describe the anatomy of left ventricle (LV) and right ventricle (RV).

The Left Ventricle

The Shape

The LV resembles an ellipsoid of revolution with its long axis directed from the base to the apex. All three noninvasive imaging techniques show this ellipsoidal geometry with cross-sections parallel to the long axis (meridian sections). Conversely, short axis cross-sections from the base to the apex reveal a circular geometry. Consequently, the interventricular septum is curved with the concavity toward the LV (Fig. 6.1). Differences also exist in the thickness of the musculature of the ventricular wall: in the normal individual the LV free wall is the thickest (12–14 mm) at the cardiac base and gradually decreases toward the apex. At the very tip of the apex the wall thickness is as thin as 2 mm (Fig. 6.2).

F. F. Faletra (✉) · L. A. Leo · V. L. Paiocchi · S. A. Schlossbauer
Non-invasive Cardiovascular Imaging Department, Fondazione
Cardiocentro Ticino, Lugano, Switzerland
e-mail: Francesco.Faletra@cardiocentro.org;
lauraanna.leo@cardiocentro.org; vera.paiocchi@cardiocentro.org;
susanne.schlossbauer@cardiocentro.org

G. Pedrazzini · T. Moccetti
Cardiology Department, Fondazione Cardiocentro Ticino,
Lugano, Switzerland
e-mail: giovanni.pedrazzini@cardiocentro.org;
tiziano.moccetti@cardiocentro.org

S. Y. Ho
Royal Brompton Hospital, Sydney Street, London, UK
e-mail: yen.ho@imperial.ac.uk

Inlet, Apical Trabeculated, and Outlet Components

The left ventricle can be divided empirically into an inlet, an apical trabeculated, and an outlet component, although well-demarcated anatomic boundaries between these three regions do not exist. Furthermore, trabeculations (muscle bundles) are not strictly limited to the apical component. Only the smooth wall of the upper part of the septum, beneath the aortic valve, is devoid of trabeculations, while the *inlet* component contains the mitral valve, chordae tendineae, and papillary muscles (PMs), and extends from the mitral hinge line to the attachment of papillary muscles. This component may present with a fairly smooth wall.

The *apical* component is characterized by fine trabeculations—thin muscular bundles that arise from compact myocardium. Not infrequently, finer strands known as false tendons extend from the septal surface, crossing the cavity to insert into the PMs and the free wall. The trabeculated component of LV roughly comprises one third of the LV but both extensions and lengths of the trabeculae into the LV cavity are highly variable among individuals.

Extensive trabeculations are, in fact, frequently found in healthy individuals. The presence of highly trabeculated LV, though, in the absence of any other structural heart disease, has raised concerns as to whether this is a pre-phenotypic marker of underlying structural heart disease such as myocardial non-compaction with potentially adverse outcome, or is just a normal anatomical variant. Studies with CT scan (the noninvasive imaging technique with highest spatial resolution power) have shown that extensive trabeculations reaching the criteria threshold for the diagnosis of non-compaction myocardium (i.e., transmural wall thickness of non-compaction to compact myocardium ratio > 2.3 in diastole) have been found also in normal healthy individuals (Fig. 6.3a, b). Moreover, studies with cardiac magnetic resonance have shown in asymptomatic individuals that marked extension of trabeculations in the

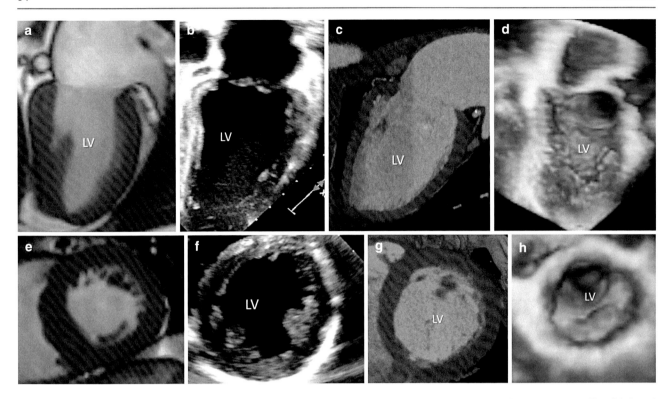

Fig. 6.1 Two-chamber long-axis views (**a**–**d**) and (**e**–**h**) short-axis view at mid-level obtained with cardiac magnetic resonance (**a**–**e**); 2D transthoracic echocardiography (**b**–**f**); computed tomography (**c**, **g**); and three-dimensional echocardiography (**d**, **h**). Showing as in long-axis sections along the meridians (**a**–**d**), the LV has an ellipsoid-shaped configuration, while in short-axis cross sections (**e**–**h**), the LV assumes a circular configuration

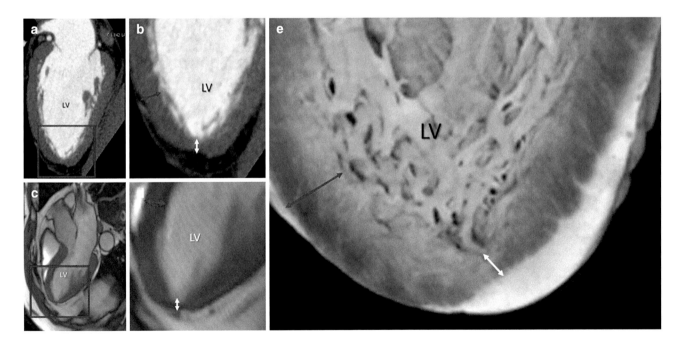

Fig. 6.2 (**a**) Computed tomography planar image in two-chamber view and (**c**) cardiac magnetic resonance in long-axis view. The areas in red boxes are magnified in (**b**) and (**d**) respectively. Both techniques beautifully visualized as the tip of apex is thinner (*white double arrow*) than the anterior (*red double arrow* in **b**) or septal (*red double arrow* in **d**) left ventricle (LV) walls. (**e**) Anatomical specimen showing the differences in thickness between the apex (*white double arrow*) and the lateral wall (*red double arrow*)

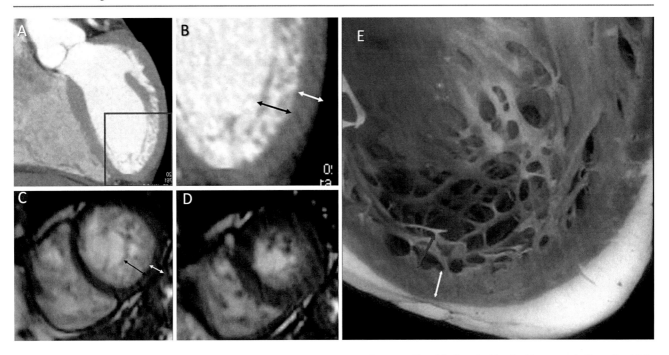

Fig. 6.3 (**a** and **b**) CT scan multiplanar imaging format in long axis view. The area in the red box is magnified in panel (**b**). Images show an extensive trabeculation in an otherwise normal individual. Black and white double-headed arrow illustrates the thickness of trabeculated and compact layers respectively (**c**, **d**). CMR cine image in short-axis view in diastole (**c**) and systole (**d**), showing an extensive trabeculation with normal contractility. *Black and white double arrows* indicate the thickness of trabeculated and compact layers respectively. (**e**) Anatomic specimen showing a highly trabeculated left ventricle in an otherwise normal heart. *Red and white double arrows* indicate the thickness of trabeculated and compact layers respectively

absence of structural heart disease, at a follow-up of as long as 10 years, is not associated with a decline of systolic function or symptoms (i.e., heart failure, ventricular arrhythmias, and systemic embolic events) (Fig. 6.3c, d). Thus, subjects with marked trabeculations in absence of any other clinical pathological aspects should not be labelled as having a potential cardiomyopathy.

Particularly interesting is the presence of highly trabeculated myocardium in athletes. Although these findings have been considered as a nonspecific epiphenomenon in response to a chronic increase in preload and afterload associated with extreme exercise, a "gray zone" and concern still persist because more or less concealed cardiomyopathy is considered one of the most common causes of effort-related sudden death in young athletes. The dilemma in differentiating between "benign" and "malignant" hypertrabeculation is due to the "ambiguous" criteria used for the diagnosis of non-compaction myocardium. Indeed, although these criteria are based on the net distinction between an outer layer where the myocardium is compacted and an inner layer formed by trabeculations and deep recesses, this latter aspect is variable in extension and in site; thus the precise point in space and in time for measuring the thickness of the two layers is still uncertain. Additional criteria (such as inappropriate increase of LV volume, reduced ejection fraction or longitudinal LV short-

ening, abnormal diastolic function, ECG anomalies, and eventually reduction of exercise capability) should be taken into account to avoid diagnosing non-compaction myocardium based merely on imaging.

The *outlet* component sustains the aortic root, but contrary to the RV outlet, which is completely muscular, the LV outlet consists of both muscular and fibrous tissues. Indeed, the posterior-medial part of the LV outlet is formed by the zone of mitral aortic continuity. This is a band of fibrous tissue that connects the hinge-line of the anterior mitral leaflets with the inter-leaflet fibrous triangle between left and non-coronary sinuses and extends between the left and right fibrous trigones. A small area of the medial aspect of LV outlet is occupied by the membranous septum. The antero-lateral aspect (almost half of the outlet circumference) is formed by musculature of ventricular septum and LV wall. Since the LV outlet component is also part of the aortic root, readers will find an additional description of the LV outlet in Chap. 2.

Papillary Muscles

Papillary muscles (PMs) are considered one of the distinctive aspects of the LV. There are usually two groups. Viewed from the atrial perspective, these two groups of

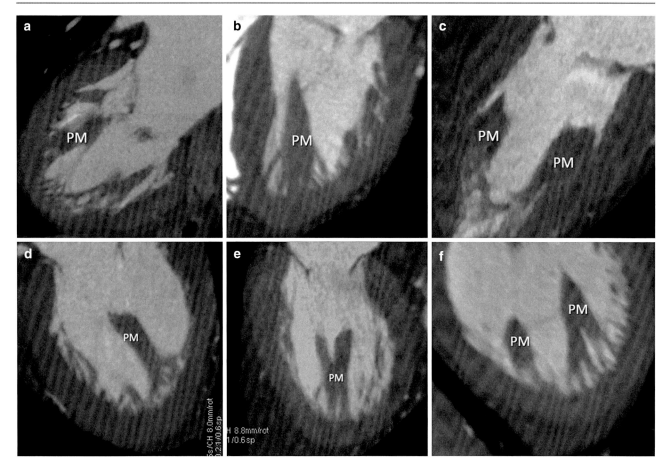

Fig. 6.4 (a–f) CT scan multiplanar images showing different shapes of papillary muscles (PM)

PMs are located near the mitral valve commissures in antero-lateral and posterior-medial position. During systole, contraction of PMs tightens chordae tendineae and prevents prolapse of mitral leaflets. The contraction of PMs is, in fact, essential for maintaining a constant distance between the tip of PMs and the area of coaptation of the mitral valve. When there is any decrease of PM's contraction, chordae tendineae become relatively too long to firmly tightening mitral leaflets at their coaptation line, and as a consequence, leaflets are free to move beyond the annular plane (leaflets prolapse), causing mitral regurgitation. PM dysfunction refers to a condition in which a PM reduces its contractile action as a result of localized ischemia. The immediate consequence is the appearance of mitral regurgitation, which may disappear if the ischemia is transitory.

PMs are usually described as two single pillar-shaped muscular protrusions with one, two, or more heads that are connected with the mitral leaflets through chordae tendineae. In reality, however, the number and shape of PMs can be extremely variable: PMs can be conical, cylindrical, broad-apexed, pyramidal, fan-shaped, flat-topped, truncated, bifurcated, and trifurcated. Finally, muscular bands

may connect the two groups of PMs, although intragroup connections are more frequent. Figure 6.4 shows different aspects of PMs as visualized by the CT.

The connections between PMs and the compact myocardium are particularly important since vessels and nerves reach the PMs through their bases. Moreover, cutting PMs during mitral valve replacement may negatively affect LV function, suggesting that the connection between the base of PMs and the wall is important in determining normal pattern of wall motion. Until few years ago, textbooks and articles depicted the PMs as having a broad base in direct connection with the compact myocardium. In 2004, Axel provided new insights in the anatomy of PMs using the CT scan. In his article, Axel showed CT images that indisputably demonstrate that the base of PMs is attached to the trabeculae rather than directly to the compact myocardium. Acquiring these "innovative" images was made possible by two conditions that are less obvious in pathological or surgical scenarios: (a) the high spatial resolution of CT technique, which has voxels as small as 0.6 mm; and (b) the time of CT images' acquisition at the end of diastole where the spaces between trabeculae that sustain the PM's body are enlarged and

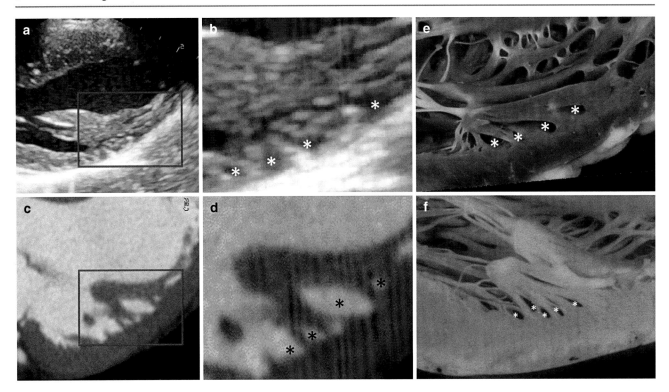

Fig. 6.5 (**a**) Detail of papillary muscle visualized with 2D echocardiography (**a**) and CT multiplanar reconstruction (**c**). The areas in the red box are magnified in (**b**) and (**d**) respectively. Images clearly show as the base of papillary muscle attached to the trabeculations rather than to the compact myocardium. *Asterisks* indicate the inter-trabeculae spaces. (**e** and **f**) Anatomic specimens showing the same architecture. *Asterisks* indicate the inter-trabeculae spaces

therefore visible (Fig. 6.5). This is an example of a noninvasive imaging technique that may help in defining fine details of anatomy that were previously disregarded or forgotten.

The arrangement between PMs and myocardium may have functional implications because this mesh-like connection with multiple points of attachment may more effectively reduce the stress on the base of PM than a pillar like attachment. Having a blood supply entering the PM body from several pathways may create a perfusion redundancy that acts as protection against ischemia.

PMs are part of the mitral valve apparatus; thus, readers also will find images and descriptions in Chap. 1.

Microstructure

Understanding LV contraction requires knowledge of the fine microstructure of the myocardium. Description at the "molecular level" of the arrangement of the myocardial fiber is beyond the scope of this chapter. Though prevalently composed by myocytes (nearly 80% of the mass of the myocardium is formed by myocytes), it must be emphasized that the myocardium contains other types of cells (endothelial cells, fibroblasts, and other connective tissue cells, mast cells and immune system-related cells, and pluri-potent "stem cells)

that interact each other and with muscular cells via a variety of paracrine, autocrine, and endocrine factors. Finally, the myocardium is permeated by a diffuse network of connective fibrils (see below), adipose tissues, arteries, veins, nerves, and lymphatics.

Myocytes

The LV myocardium consists of 2–3 billion cells called *myocytes*. The myocyte is a long thin cell of approximately of 100–120 μm in length and 20 μm in diameter and is surrounded by a membrane (sarcolemma). Each myocyte is firmly connected with surrounding cells by *intercalated disks*, either through end-to-end or side-by-side joining. The intercalated discs are part of the sarcolemma and contain two components essential for the myocardial contraction: the *gap junctions* and *desmosomes*. The gap junctions are channels between myocytes that directly link the cytoplasm of adjoining cells and provide a relatively unrestricted passage of ions. The gap junctions between myocytes form a complex three-dimensional network of anastomosing cells, a sort of *syncytium*. The *desmosomes* are a complex arrangement of proteins across two adjacent sarcolemma that anchor them together so they do not pull apart during the contraction of individual myocytes. Myocytes characteristically contain an

Sub-epicardium	Mid-wall	Sub-endocardium

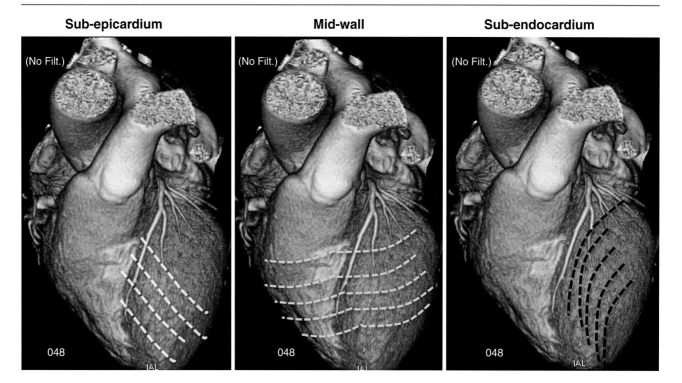

Fig. 6.6 CT scan volume rendering format with superimposed line of prevalent orientation of myofibers in sub-epicardium, mid-wall, and sub-endocardium

impressive number of mitochondria that produce high levels of ATP. In any myocyte the sarcolemma projects long, finger-like invaginations called *T-tubules* into the cytoplasm. The T-tubules join sacs or channels of *sarcoplasmic reticulum* in a way that two sacs of the reticulum are positioned laterally to a single T-tubule (the so called *triade*). This configuration is the anatomical basis of excitation-contraction: indeed, when a positively charged current is transmitted from the *neuromuscular junction* it runs down to the T-tubule. The influx of calcium activates receptors of the adjacent sacs, which initiate a release of calcium ions. Calcium ions, in turn, activate a precise cascade of events consisting of complex rearrangements of several molecules, which eventually leads to a contraction (see below).

The *myofibrils* are undoubtfully the fundamental structure of myocyte. About 80% of the sarcoplasm of myocytes is occupied by myofibrils. Myofibrils are substantially linear structures that resemble cables running parallel to the long axis of the myocytes. They are made up of millions of *sarcomeres*, the true "engines" of the contraction. The sarcomere is about 3 μm in length and each myofibril contains thousands of sarcomeres that together cover the entire length of the myofibril. The sarcomeres are connected end-to-end at the so-called *Z-line*. Each sarcomere contains thick and thin myofilaments called *myosin* and *actin* respectively, interdigitated with one another. The Z-line acts as scaffold connecting thin filaments from adjacent sarcomeres. Myosin and actin are interconnected with a series of specialized proteins

(myosin, myosin binding protein-C, titin, actin, troponin, tropomyosin, nebulin, and others) which contributes to the shortening and lengthening of the sarcomere. The capability of sarcomeres for shortening and elongating rhythmically occurs when these parallel thick and thin filaments slide with each other thanks to "cross bridges" that form in presence of ATP. In other words, the filaments of actin protein form the "ladder" along which the filaments of myosin "climb" to generate motion. These small "engines" have the capability of shortening up to 30–35%. Under physiological conditions, however, a shortening of only 10–20% is necessary (Figs. 6.6 and 6.7).

The Extracellular Matrix

The *extracellular matrix* is another fundamental component of the myocardial structure. A fine network of collagen fibers called *endomysium* wraps each myocyte, reinforces the role of intercalated discs in binding myocytes to one another, thus preventing the slippage between cells, and acts in such a way that it synchronizes the transmission force between myocytes. The *perimysium* is a more robust and thicker network of connective fibers that groups thousands of myocytes into the so-called *myofibers*. Moreover, lateral connective strands anchor myofibers to each other, preventing a malalignment. Blood and lymphatic vessels, and fibers of the conduction system that serve the myocytes, run in the perimysial space

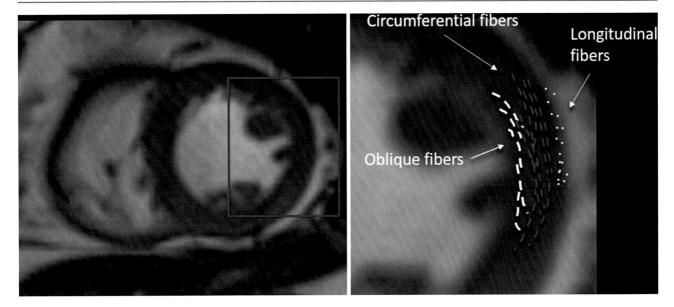

Fig. 6.7 CMR image in short-axis view. The area in the red box is magnified to the right. Directional lines of myofibers are depicted in white in the sub-endocardium, in red in the mid-wall, and in yellow in the sub-epicardium

between myofibers. A perimysial sheet allows the myofibers to slide alongside one another during the cardiac cycle (see below). Finally, myofibers are packed together by the *epimysium*, which surrounds the entire myocardial mass.

Relation Between Myocardial Structure and Function

The relationship between myocardial structure and myocardial function has been debated for several decades, if not centuries. Several hypotheses have been described, ranging from laminar sheets, layered fibers, complex nested syncytium, to a unique band arrangement organized in two distinct helicoids. Nowadays, most anatomists and physiologists agree that the ventricular mass is arranged on the basis on an interweaving network of myofibers. Moreover, two helical fibers arrangements have been recognized: a right-handed helical arrangement that takes place in the subendocardial region with an angulation respect to the longitudinal axes of +60°, and a left-handed helical configuration in subepicardial regions (−60°). Thus, the majority of subepicardial myocardial fibers overlap those of subepicardium with an angle of 120°. In the subepicardium, myocardial and in papillary muscles fibers may also run vertically. This counter-directional arrangement of myocardial fibers maintains stability and minimizes energy expenditure. At mid-wall, halfway between epicardium and endocardium, myocardial fibers lie in the circumferential plane aligned with short axis sections and perpendicular to long axis planes. It must be said that these three layers are not at all separated by cleavage planes since myofibers of one layer are interconnected

with myofibers of an adjacent layer. Thus, the overall histological picture is that of a meshwork.

Recent advances in cardiac magnetic resonance allow direct visualization of the myocardial fiber architecture using diffusion tensor imaging. This novel method has emerged as the gold standard for "nondestructive" reconstruction of fibers orientation (in opposite to "destructive" studies when dissections of anatomic specimens are used). This is based on the principle that the main orientation of the fibers parallels the diffusion of water molecules, which causes a signal attenuation in the presence of a magnetic field. This method allows the capture of impressive images of the actual arrangement of fibers in vivo.

Thickening, Longitudinal Shortening, and Torsion

The LV is capable of ejecting during exercise more than 100 mL of blood (which is viscous liquid) against over 200 mmHg, and then receiving the same quantity at less 10 mmHg and in less than 100 ms. This incredible performance is possible because during systole the LV myocardium thickens radially, shortens along meridians, and the apex twists relative to the base.

Ventricular *wall thickening* is an important mechanism for systolic ejection, accounting for 25–50% of stroke volume. Myocardial fibers, myocytes, myofibrils, and sarcomeres have an "elongated" appearance. It is therefore intuitive to suppose that they are structured to shorten along their major axis. In a cascade of events, shortening of the sarcomere should cause shortening of the fibril and, subsequently, a shortening of the myocytes and myocardial fibers. However, since myocardial fibers are arranged almost parallel to the endo, meso, and epicardial surfaces of the LV, the wall thickening must take place not only because fibers shorten but also because they "thicken."

During systole the ejection fraction of LV is 50–70%, and the increase in wall thickness is 30–50%. Both vastly exceed sarcomere thickening that is only 10%.How can the wall thickness increase by 30%, while the fibers thickening only 10%? Indeed, increase in cell diameter (thickening) as myocytes shorten, would contribute only about one fifth of the thickening of the wall. Moreover, while the shortening of the fibers is substantially the same from the epicardium to the endocardium and from the apex to the base, the parietal thickening is greater in the inner than in the outer layers.

There is an almost universal agreement among anatomists that the ventricular myocardium has a laminar organization in which myocytes are grouped into branching layers (three to six cells thick) surrounded by an extensive perimysial collagen network and separated by sheet cleavage planes.

Though significant regional variations in the organization of the laminae may exist, this structure provides a rational explanation between arrangement of myocytes and systolic wall thickening. Indeed, it can be observed that these myocardial *laminae* assume in diastole an oblique direction from top to bottom and from the outside toward the inside. In systole, the laminae slide one on the other along the cleavage planes, assuming a direction more perpendicular to the long axis of the ventricle. This change of direction is probably determined by the contraction of the longitudinal fibers present in the subepicardium and subendocardium. Thus, the thickening of the wall does not take place only because millions of fibers shorten and thicken, but also because of a rearrangement of myocardial laminae: in systole the laminae are arranged more "perpendicular" with respect to the long axis of the ventricle, and in this way they increase the wall thickness. The laminar myocardial structure with sheets of myocytes separated by cleavage planes seem to be appositely designed for a radial thickening. Obviously, the opposite occurs in diastole (Fig. 6.8).

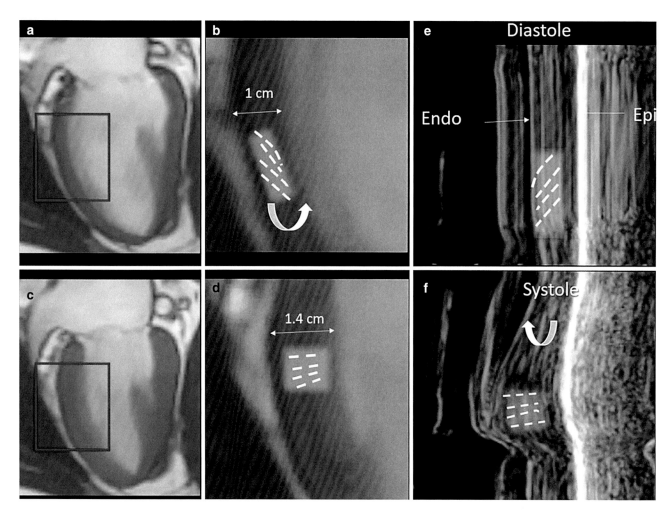

Fig. 6.8 CMR images in long-axis view in diastole (**a**) and systole (**c**). The areas in the red boxes are magnified in (**b**) and (**d**) respectively. The superimposed dotted lines show the "laminae" that in diastole assume an oblique direction from top to bottom and from the outside toward the inside. In systole the laminae slide one on the other along the cleavage planes, assuming a direction more perpendicular to the long axis of the ventricle. *Curved arrow* marks the direction of the motion. (**e–f**) M-Mode echocardiography showing the radial thickening of the posterior wall in one point. *Dotted lines* represent the disposition of laminae in diastole (upper half of the figure) and in systole (see text)

Longitudinal shortening occurs because of contraction of sub-endocardial and sub-epicardial oblique/longitudinal fibers. Because the apex is firmly attached to the diaphragm, the longitudinal shortening leads to the descent of the atrioventricular and aortic valve planes (Fig. 6.9). It is interesting to note that the aortic and mitral translation toward and away from the LV apex determines a passive displacement of a column of blood across the valves. The diastolic translation of mitral annulus away from the apex, for example, promotes LV filling by displacing the column of blood initially present in left atrium to underneath the mitral leaflets. In systole, the translation of mitral plane toward the apex enlarges the left atrium with a consequent drop in atrial pressure. This atrial "vacuum" promotes the pulmonary venous return. In the absence of longitudinal shortening, as occurs in hypertrophic or infiltrative cardiomyopathies, the left atrium does not enlarge, and the left atrial pressure remains high, preventing a regular inflow of blood from the pulmonary veins with increase of pulmonary capillary pressure and consequent transudation into the interstitial space. This mechanism causes symptoms of heart failure. Of note, this may occur in the presence of preserved ejection fraction since the systolic contraction may be maintained by the radial thickening, the so-called "heart failure with preserved ejection fraction." On the other hand, the motion of the aortic root toward the apex displaces the column of blood from the outflow tract to the aorta, increasing the systolic stroke volume.

Twist, untwist, rotation, torsion—these terms have been used in the literature to describe systolic rotation and diastolic reverse rotation of the LV base and apex as viewed from the apex. In other words, the LV has a "wringing" motion (Fig. 6.9).

The contraction of subendocardial myofibers should rotate the apex in opposite directions. The outer subepicardial layers dominate the overall direction of rotation; however, myocardial activation occurs first in the subendocardial layers, which therefore shorten earlier, stretching the subepicardial layers during the isovolumetric phase, causing a brief LV un-twist. During the ejection period, the subepicardial layers dominate the direction of the rotation. Of note is the role of the myocardial connective network: during systole, myocardial contraction stretches the connective fibrils. The stored energy is released during diastole, facilitating a diastolic recoil. LV mechanics can be assessed non-invasively using echocardiography (in particular, speckle tracking) and cardiac magnetic resonance using tissue tagging.

The Role of Blood

LV is considered as a pressure generator. Thinking of the LV as a "hydraulic pump" derives from the concept that the blood is an inert, amorphous liquid that must be pushed "by force" into the circulation. The concept of the heart as a generator of pressure in the cardiological community has been imposed by the fact that most of our knowledge in terms of the physiology of the cardiovascular system is essentially derived from the measurement of hemodynamic pressure curves. As mentioned, the singular arrangement of myocytes in laminae and helical configuration allows a complex contraction where radial thickening, longitudinal shortening, and apical twisting act together for generating a systolic pressure to push the blood through arterial vessels. However, there is still ongoing debate on the "energetic sustainability" of the myocardium in doing this work. Indeed, 300 g of muscular tissue must be able to "push" thousands of liters of inert blood every day (with a viscosity five times greater than that of water) through billions of arterioles and capillaries (whose last dimensions are not greater than the diameter of the erythrocytes). Moreover, the anatomy of the ventricular cavity would appear to be not completely suitable for being a "generator" of pressure. The apex, for example, has a considerably thinner wall than the base and is therefore more subject to the action of intraventricular pressure (Fig. 6.10).

The hypothesis of an additional source of energy generated directly by the blood itself (which then is no longer an inert liquid) is fascinating. In the fetal period when the heart is still a tube and does not generate pressure, the blood advances like a liquid cylinder rotating with a spiral movement along the axis of advancement. The propulsion force is given by the movement of the blood itself, which advances by virtue of its rotary movement (like a vortex). In the early stages of development, the blood rotating in the cardiac cavity would transfer its momentum (i.e., mass × speed) to the muscle. In this way, the blood momentum would combine with that of the heart, favoring rotation and propulsion. In other words, the spiraling structure and movement of the heart would be the consequence of the inherent spiraling movement of the blood, and not vice versa. This is a general tendency of liquids that, in nature, tend to move in a spiral way (just see how the water goes down the sink to reach the drain). The heart with its contraction would favor and perpetuate this rotational movement by minimizing energy expenditure. It is possible that the structure of the cardiovascular system has specialized in the course of millions of years to obtain the maximum benefit from this propensity of liquids (including blood) to flow in a spiral-like manner.

A sort of "electronic cast" can be obtained with CT making transparent the myocardium and increasing the opacity of intracavitary contrast. These electronic casts characteristically show a helical disposition of trabeculations. Whether arrangement is "sculptured" by the spiral movement of the blood is unknown (Fig. 6.11).

The Right Ventricle

In 1943 Star et al. noted that major destruction of the right ventricle causes only minimal changes in venous and arterial pressure. Similar studies later confirmed that extensive dam-

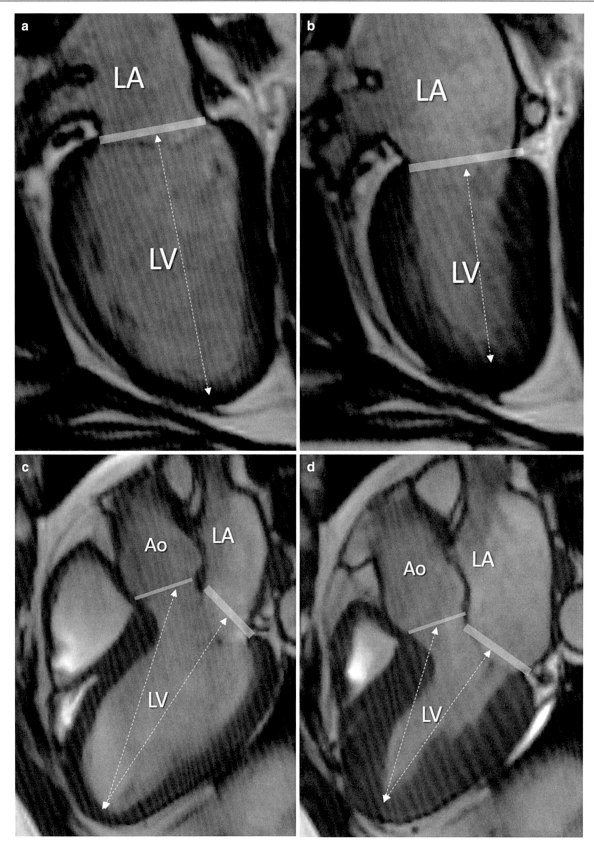

Fig. 6.9 Longitudinal shorting assessed by CMR in two chamber view (a, b) and long-axis view (c, d). Because the apex is stationary, the longitudinal shortening produces the atrio-ventricular (*thick line*) and aortic (*thin line*) planes to descend toward the apex. *Dotted double arrowlines* mark the distance between mitral and aortic planes and the apex in diastole (a, c) and in systole (b, d)

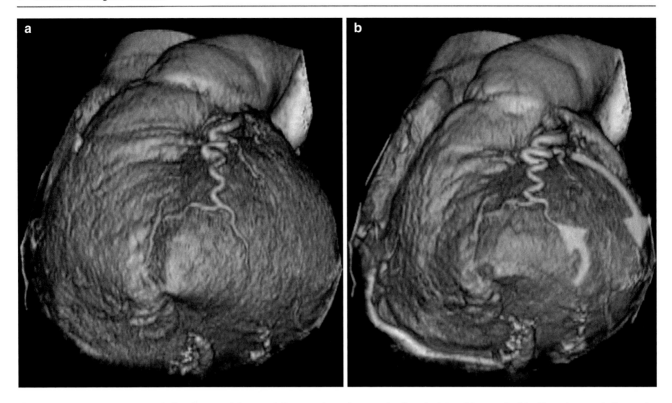

Fig. 6.10 CT scan volume-rendering format of the ventricles seen from the apex in diastole (**a**) and in systole (**b**). *Curved arrow* indicates the counterclockwise rotation of the apex and the clockwise rotation of the base

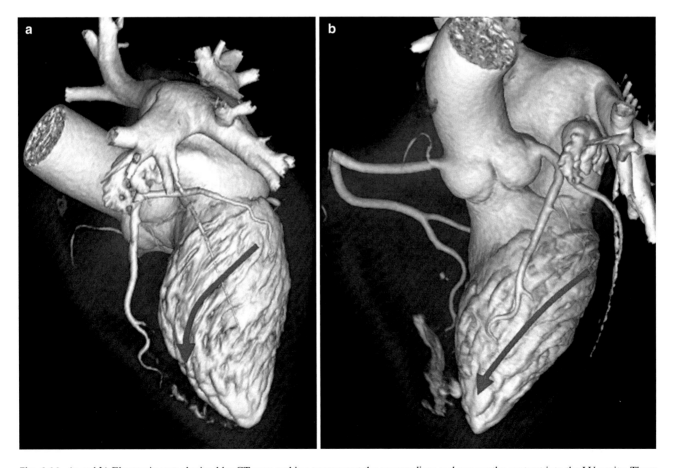

Fig. 6.11 (**a** and **b**) Electronic cast obtained by CT scan making transparent the myocardium and opaque the contrast into the LV cavity. These casts show a helical arrangement of trabeculations (*curved red arrows*)

age of RV does not produce right heart failure and venous congestion. Thus, in the middle of the nineteenth century, the leading opinion was that a normal contractile RV wall is not necessary for the maintenance of a "normal circulation." Today we know that, in case of a failure of RV, contraction of the LV may indeed support the circulation, though for a limited period of time, with the contraction of interventricular septum (see below). The belief that the RV had substantially negligible clinical relevance was further reinforced by the use of Fontan surgical procedure in patients with tricuspid atresia and rudimentary RV or other so-called univentricular hearts. The surgical intervention consists of diverting the venous blood from inferior and superior vena cava to the pulmonary arteries by creating a total cavo-to-pulmonary arterial communication that completely excludes the RV from the circulation.

Like the tricuspid valve, the RV therefore became a "forgotten" chamber and was disregarded by the cardiology community for decades. Only a couple of decades ago accumulating evidence emphasized the relevance of RV in almost any cardiac scenarios, for both its clinical impact and its prognostic implications. Herein we present an update of the normal RV anatomy, as we believe that a detailed knowledge of RV anatomy is an indispensable prerequisite to understand RV abnormalities, and is also valuable for electrophysiologists during their invasive procedures and device implantations. Finally, we conclude the chapter by describing the anatomy of the pulmonary valve.

Location and Shape of the RV

Situated directly behind the sternum and anterior to LV, the RV is a thin-walled crescent-shaped ventricular chamber (Fig. 6.12).

From an anterior-posterior perspective the RV appears to have a triangular/trapezoidal shaped aspect. Along its transverse axis the RV curves antero-superiorly, wrapping around the LV (Fig. 6.13). This complex anatomy cannot be fitted to simple geometric models, and this is the major limitation for understanding RV volume and function when it is measured in two-dimensional tomographic views.

This shape, as well as the fact that the two ventricles share the interventricular septum, pericardium, and myofibers (especially their superficial layers) explain the phenomenon of the "interdependence" of the ventricles. Indeed, while the RV has little or no effect on the LV contraction, roughly 30% of the contractile energy of the RV is generated by the LV which, through the septal contraction, contributes significantly to RV pressure generation.

In the normal adult heart, the wall of the RV is considerably thinner than that of the left ventricle, ranging from 3 to 7 mm, but being as thin as 1.5 mm at the tip of the apex. The RV appears therefore quite vulnerable to perforation by catheters and pacemaker leads positioned near the apex (Fig. 6.14b). Accordingly, the RV mass is about one-sixtieth that of LV mass. Nevertheless, in normal conditions, the RV is perfectly adequate for ejecting blood in a low impedance pulmonary vasculature. Owing to its thinner wall, the RV has a greater compliance than the LV. Because of these anatomical characteristics, it is perfectly comprehensible that the RV tolerates volume overload better than pressure overload (Fig. 6.14).

Inlet, Apical Trabeculated, and Outlet

In the normally developed RV, with normal atrioventricular and ventriculoarterial concordance and normal tricuspid and pulmonary valves, the RV can be divided into three major regions: inlet, apical, and outlet, although no clear anatomical demarcations can be seen between these parts (Fig. 6.15a). The inflow/outflow axis angle of the RV is significantly wider than that of LV. This anatomical architecture requires that the right outflow tract must contribute to the overall RV ejection fraction (see below) (Fig. 6.15b). Interestingly, the RV outflow tract has a different embryological origin than the remaining RV myocardium.

The *inlet component* surrounds and supports the tricuspid valve and its subvalvular apparatus extending from the hinge line of tricuspid valve up to the insertion of papillary muscles (Fig. 6.15a). The *apical component* is characterized by trabeculations that are thicker than the counterpart LV trabeculations. These coarse trabeculations may help to distinguish the "morphological" RV from the morphological LV irrespective of the position of the chamber within the heart.

The *outlet component* or infundibulum consists of a muscular "freestanding" tube-like portion, free of trabeculations, which supports the pulmonary valve. It accounts for nearly 20% of the right volume. The posterior aspect of the RV outlet is formed by the supraventricular crest (see below). Interestingly, the RV outlet is separated from the aorta by a cleavage plane filled with epicardial fat. Thus, the RV outlet can be removed surgically without entering in the LV cavity (Fig. 6.16).

This particular anatomical configuration allows retrieval of the patient's own pulmonary valve with its muscle sleeve to replace the patient's diseased aortic valve in the Ross procedure. The pulmonary valve is then replaced with a pulmonary allograft. This is the procedure of choice in children and infants with aortic valve disease.

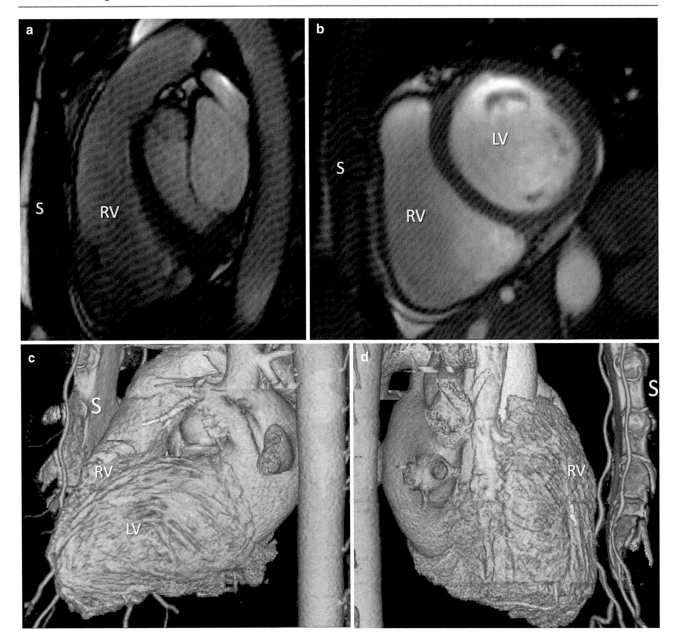

Fig. 6.12 CMR in longitudinal (**a**) and cross-sectional (**b**) view and CT electronic casts (**c** and **d**) in two different perspectives showing the right ventricle (RV) anterior to left ventricle (LV) located just behind the sternum (S)

Specific Anatomic Structures

Within the RV cavity three structures are peculiar to the RV: the supraventricular crest, the septomarginal trabeculation, and the moderator band.

The supraventricular crest is a prominent muscular structure that forms the posterior wall of the RV outlet and separates the inlet from the outlet components of RV. Indeed, contrary to the left side where the aortic and mitral valves are adjacent to each other and connected by a fibrous band (*see* Chap. 1), the

tricuspid and pulmonary valves are widely separated by this muscular wall. In cross-section at its septal origin, the supraventricular crest looks like a semilunar ridge with the origin of the right coronary artery on its epicardial aspect. Seen from an external perspective it is clear that it is an infolding of the RV wall (the ventricular-infundibular fold) that extends from its septal origin, accommodating the aortic root, and tapers as it extends parietally. As mentioned, a space (often virtual) filled by a leaf of epicardial fat separates the supraventricular crest (and the infundibulum) from the aorta (Fig. 6.17).

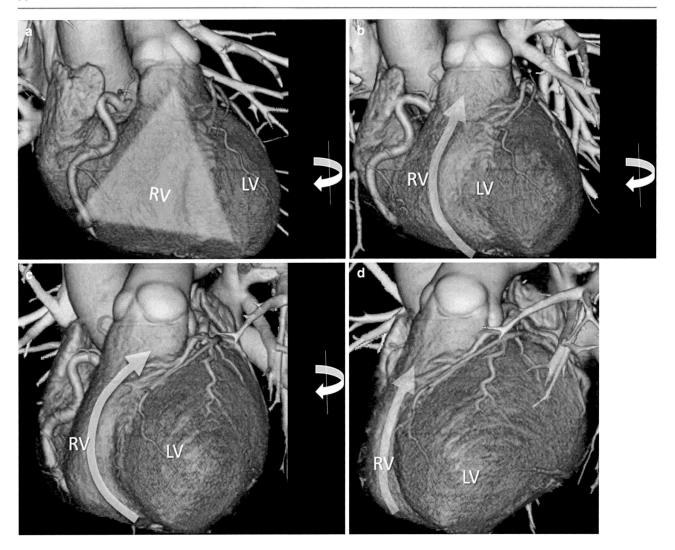

Fig. 6.13 (**a–d**) CT scan volume rendering showing as in antero-posterior perspective (**a**) the RV has a triangle-shaped aspect. By rotating the image from right to left around the y-axis (*curved arrow*), it appears that the RV wraps around the LV (*curved arrows*)

The term *septomarginal trabecula* (SMT) was first use in 1913 by Tandler, who noted that this muscular band was attached proximally to the septum and distally to the margin of RV. Indeed, the SMT is a muscular column protruding from the septal surface beginning below the supraventricular crest and continues toward the anterolateral wall of the RV joining, through the moderator band (see below), the base of anterior papillary muscle (see also Chap. 3 on the tricuspid valve).

While superiorly the SMT bifurcates in two arms that embrace the ventriculo-infundibular fold forming the supraventricular crest, the column-like body extends toward the ventricular apex, where it gives origin to the *moderator band* (MB).

The MB takes its name as a result of a supposition that it may control or "moderate" an excessive dilation of the RV when too much blood fills it. Indeed, it has a characteristic course crossing the right ventricular cavity and ends at the base of anterior papillary muscle, where it attaches to the RV free wall.

Interestingly, the right bundle branch of the conducting system runs through the subendocardium of the SMT and the MB carries a significant sub-branch across the RV cavity to the parietal RV wall. The SMT, the moderator band, and the anterior papillary muscle form a "U-shaped" protrusion into the RV cavity that separates the inflow from the outflow. Abnormal hypertrophy of these structures may potentially lead to an intracavitary obstruction dividing the RV into two chambers, one proximal at high pressure and one distal at low pressure (double-chambered RV) (Fig. 6.18).

Microstructure

Normal myocytes of RV appear smaller than the LV myocytes, while the RV contains more extracellular matrix in terms of collagen fibers. Characteristically, while the LV myocardium has three distinct layers, anatomical dissections of the RV reveal only two layers: the subepicardial

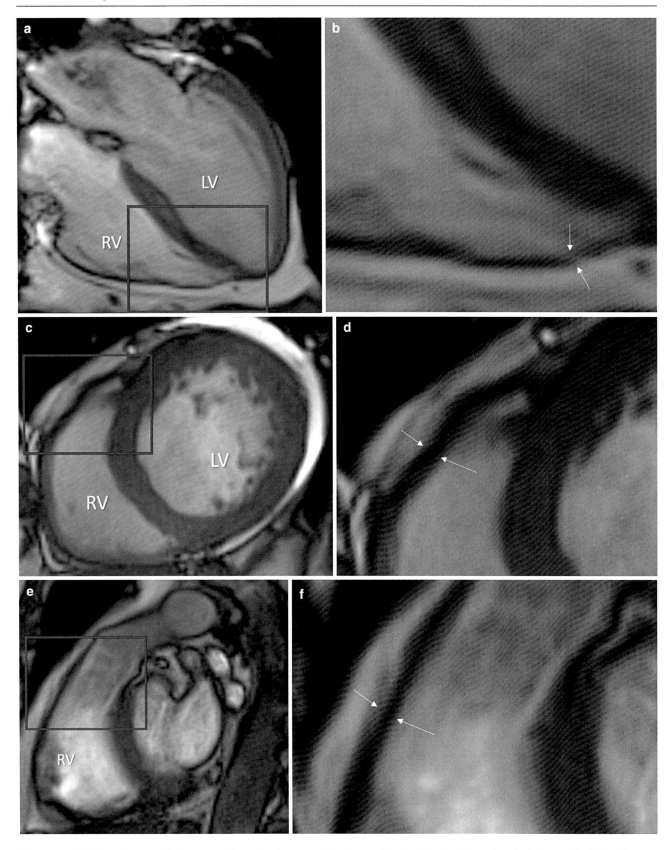

Fig. 6.14 CMR four-chamber (**a**), short axis (**c**), and outflow tract (**e**) sections of the right ventricle (RV). The areas in red boxes are magnified in (**b**), (**d**), and (**f**), respectively. The images show the RV wall (*arrows*) is significantly thinner than the left ventricle (LV) wall, especially at the apex (**b**)

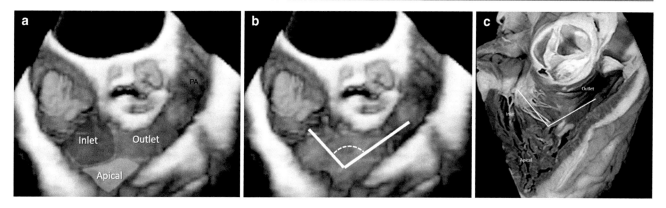

Fig. 6.15 3D TEE (**a**) showing the three regions of the right ventricle (inlet, apical, and outlet marked with red, yellow, and blue respectively) and the angle between inlet and outlet (**b**). (**c**) The corresponding anatomical specimen

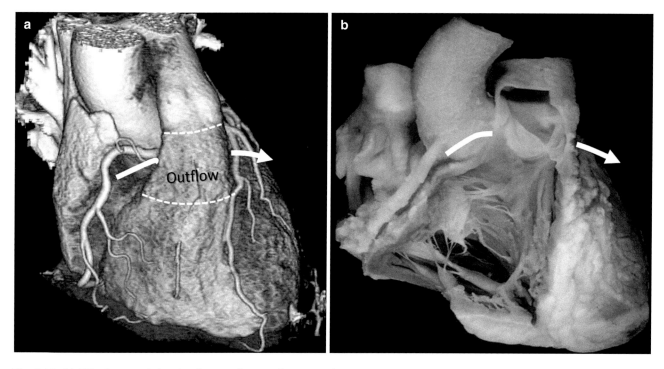

Fig. 6.16 (**a**) CT volume rendering showing as a cleavage plane (*curved arrow*), separates the RV outflow tract from the aorta and left ventricle. (**b**) The corresponding anatomical specimen

layer formed by oblique fibers almost parallel to the atrio-ventricular groove, and the subendocardial layer where fibers are preferentially arranged in an oblique fashion (Fig. 6.18).

The Subvalvular Apparatus

Although classically the PMs of the right ventricle have been described as comprising three blocks (septal, anterior, and inferior [or posterior]), this is not always the case. Indeed, the RV PMs are highly variable in number, position, and size. The anterior PM is quite large, frequently unique or

bifid. It is consistently found in anatomic specimens. The inferior PM usually consists of two or three thin PMs originating from the inferior and posterior RV wall. Characteristically, several chordae tendineae attach to the septal leaflet and originate directly from the septal wall. But at the commissure between septal and anterior leaflets, the fan-shaped commissural cord is attached to a septal PM, which is better known as the medial/conal PM or muscle of Lancisi. Originating from the posterior limb of the SMT, it is small and sometimes inconspicuous (see Chap. 3 on the tricuspid valve). As for the left PMs, the right PMs do not attach directly to the compact myocardium but originate from the trabeculations.

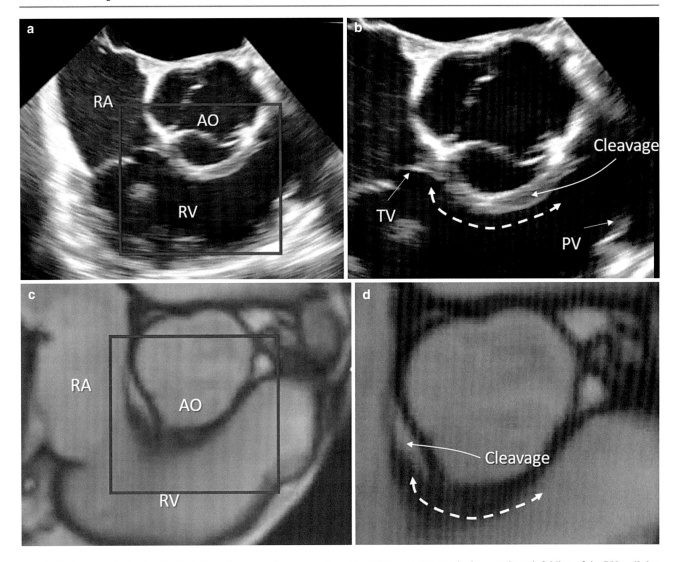

Fig. 6.17 Images obtained with 2D TEE (**a**) and cardiac magnetic resonance (**c**). The areas in red boxes are magnified in (**b**) and (**d**) respectively. The double arrows mark the extension of the supraventricular crest from the tricuspid to the pulmonary valve. Images clearly show that the supraventricular crest is an infolding of the RV wall that accommodates the aortic root. The supraventricular crest is separated from the aortic root by a cleavage plane filled by epicardial fat

Pattern of RV Contraction

Knowledge of RV function is still incomplete and certainly behind what we know about the LV. Herein, we present knowledge on the pattern of RV contraction based on current literature. RV contraction consists of three main types: longitudinal shortening, radial shortening, and contraction of LV septum. In contrast to the left ventricle, twisting and rotation motion of the RV are less consistently documented and appear to be less relevant for RV contraction and stroke volume. Longitudinal shortening is due to the longitudinal fibers located on the subendocardial layer and draws the tricuspid and pulmonary valve planes toward the apex. The longitudinal shortening appears to be a major contributor of RV stroke

volume, accounting for approximately 75% of right ventricular stroke volume (Fig. 6.19a). The radial shortening consists of the inward movement of the free wall of RV, mainly due to shortening of subepicardial fibers (Fig. 6.19b). Importantly, the interventricular septum contributes to RV contraction (the systolic interdependence). The contraction of LV, in fact, produces a bulging of the interventricular septum into the RV and simultaneously stretches the free wall of the RV over the septum; both mechanisms thus promote the inward motion of the RV wall, contributing to the reduction of the RV cavity (Fig. 6.19b).

As mentioned, the RV ventricle may be divided into inlet, apical, and outlet. These parts are completely integrated with each other, and many observers consider the RV as a single

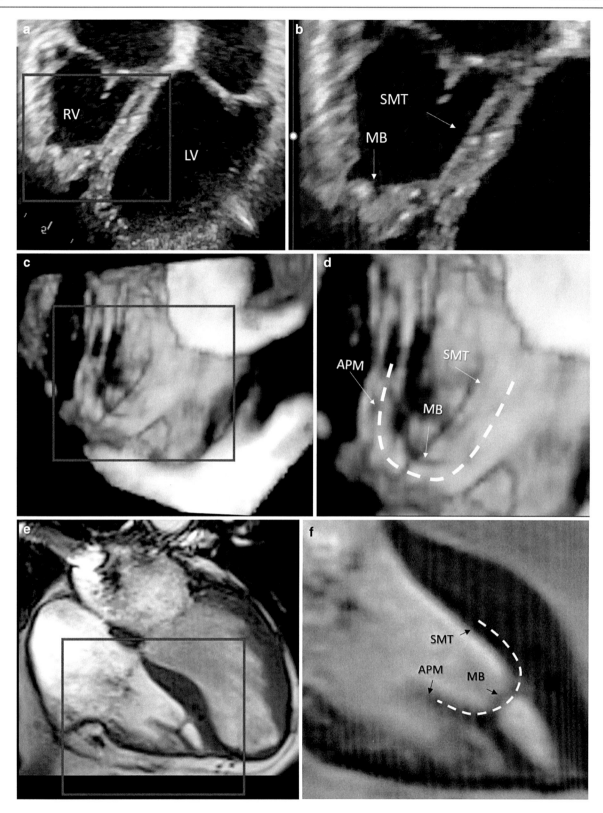

Fig. 6.18 (a) 2D transthoracic echocardiography four-chamber view. The area into the red box is magnified in (b). Images show the septo-marginal trabecula (SMT) in continuity with the moderator band. (c) 3D TEE showing the RV cavity. The area in the red box is magnified in (d). 3D images clearly show the continuity between the SMT, MB, and anterior papillary muscle (AMP). (e) CMR four-chamber view. The area in the red box is magnified in (f). This complex forms a "U-shaped" entity (curved dotted line), that separates the inflow from the outflow (see text)

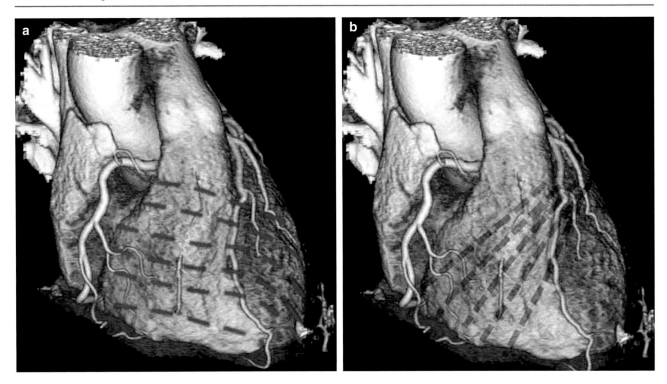

Fig. 6.19 (a) CT volume-rendering images showing the RV fibers of subepicardial layer (*red thick dotted line*) and the RV fibers of subendocardial layer (**b**, black dotted line) (see text)

functional unit. However, the inlet and outlet components may also be considered as distinct chambers given their different embryological origins. Moreover, activation of the outlet occurs relatively late in systole, being the last component of RV to be activated. Thus, regional differences in the time of contraction may be expected. Indeed, a "peristalsis-like" motion theory postulates that the RV inlet contractions occurs 20–40 ms before the RV outflow contraction. This characteristic pattern allows a coordinated movement of the column of flow from the inlet to the outlet, with the blood moving toward the RV outflow a few milliseconds before it contracts. In several reports this peristalsis was documented in cross-sections but not in longitudinal sections. RV focal systolic outpouching in the apical-lateral wall of the RV is rather common in normal subjects and is closely associated with moderator band insertions. This regional wall motion "abnormality," when occurring in isolation, should be considered a common variant of normal RV pattern of contraction.

The Pulmonary Root

Often the term "pulmonary valve"implies the pulmonary leaflets only (i.e., the thin leaves of connective/elastic tissue that open and close, following the pressure gradient between pulmonary artery and RV). In this chapter we use the term "pulmonary root" for the whole proximal segment of the pul-

monary trunk and its adjoining immediate RV outlet that supports the valvular leaflets. In fact, the pulmonary root comprises the sinotubular junction, the pulmonary sinuses, leaflets, interleaflet triangles, and the ventriculoarterial junction (see below).

2D TTE is the primary imaging technique for the assessment of the normal and abnormal anatomy of the pulmonary valve. However, given its retrosternal location and the tomographic nature of the 2DTTE, simultaneously visualizing the three pulmonary leaflets is very difficult, if not impossible. Also, 2D TEE is not the ideal modality because the PV is the most anterior valve, and therefore the most distant valve from the esophagus. 3D TEE may have the potential to visualize the three pulmonary leaflets from an "en face" perspective. However, the thinness of the leaflets and their position almost parallel to the ultrasound beam combine to produce large dropout artifacts that do not allow acquisition of images of the leaflets in their entirety in "en face" perspective, unlike for aortic leaflets, where dropout artifacts are less pronounced (*see* Chap. 2).

CMR may visualize pulmonary leaflets, but their rapid motion and thinness cause blurring artifacts that reduce the quality of CMR images (Fig. 6.20).

CT is able to visualize pulmonary leaflets and its high spatial resolution produces the clearest images of the valve. Unfortunately, its temporal resolution is at best 15 images per second using retrospective imaging acquisition, which is not ideal for appreciating the rapid motion of leaflets.

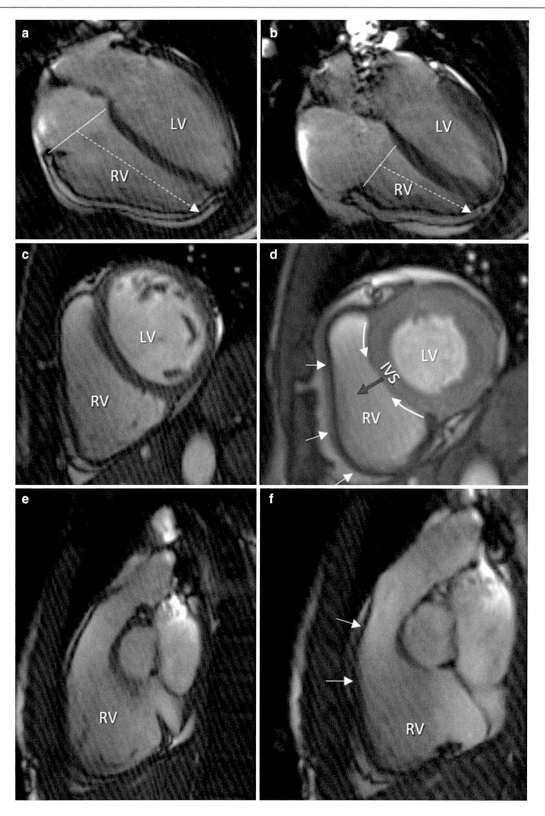

Fig. 6.20 CMR images in four-chamber (**a** and **b**), short-axis view (**c** and **d**) and long-axis views (**e** and **f**), showing the different patterns of contraction of right ventricle (RV). The longitudinal shortening is best appreciated in four-chamber view. The white line indicates the tricuspid annular plane, while the arrow indicates the excursion of the plane towards the apex showing the amount of longitudinal shortening. The radial shortening is better appreciated in short axis view (**c**, **d**). The small arrows indicate the inward motion of the free lateral wall. The red arrow indicates the bulging of interventricular septum (IVS) and the curved arrows indicate the contraction which stretches the free RV wall, contributing to this inward motion. (**e** and **f**) The inward motion of RV outlet (*arrows*). *LV* left ventricle

Moreover, retrospective acquisition causes a significant increase in radiation exposure. Thus, none of the noninvasive imaging techniques is the ideal technique for obtaining consistently good images of pulmonary leaflets. Nevertheless, CT volume-rendering modality may produce exquisite images of the shape of the pulmonary root and inter-leaflet triangles, especially when the acquisition is taken when the contrast is still in the RV cavity, whereas in patients with a favorable transesophageal echocardiographic window, the relatively high spatial (1 mm) and temporal (50 frame/s) resolution permit clear images of pulmonary leaflets for appreciating their motion.

Anatomy

Despite the different pressures, the anatomy of the pulmonary root is almost identical to the aortic root. Indeed, as in the aortic root, it comprises three leaflets, three sinuses of Valsalva, a crown-shaped annulus, commissures, and inter-leaflet fibrous triangles. The pulmonary root is the terminal part of the right ventricular outflow tract and supports pulmonary leaflets. Because in the normal individual the hemodynamic forces in the pulmonary circulation are nearly one fifth of that of systemic circulation, generally, all the components of the pulmonary root are thinner and more delicate and flexible than the aortic counterpart. The *sinu-tubular junction* delimits the pulmonary root from the tubular pulmonary trunk. This junction is not as well-defined as in the left counterpart: a true circular ridge is rarely found—more often it is possible to discern only a line separating the

slightly thinner wall of the sinuses from the thicker wall of the pulmonary trunk.

The *pulmonary leaflets* have the same "bird's nest" shape as the aortic leaflets, and analogous to the architecture of the aortic leaflets, have a crown-shaped insertion (hingeline) that crosses the ventriculo-arterial junction on the pulmonary wall. Their cranial points, the commissures, reach the sinutubular junction, while the most caudal points, the nadirs, are inserted into musculature of the infundibulum. Two leaflets face the right and left aortic leaflets and take the name of right and left leaflets. The third leaflet (the non-facing leaflet), being the most anterior, usually takes the name of anterior leaflet.

The *ventriculo-arterial junction* is the border between the fibro-elastic wall of the vessel (including its sinuses) and the muscular tissue of the infundibulum. Three *interleaflet triangles* arise from the ventriculo-arterial junction up to the sinutubular junction. These triangles are segments of fibrous tissue between the hingelines of adjacent leaflets. Although located at the base of the pulmonary trunk, they are incorporated in the RV when the valve leaflets are in closed position. Interestingly, the nadirs of the pulmonary leaflets cross the ventriculo-arterial junction. In other words, the pulmonary sinuses consist of, distally, the fibro-elastic tissue of arterial wall, and proximally, RV myocardium (Fig. 6.21). Thus, small segments of muscular RV outflow tract are enclosed within the three pulmonary sinuses. These may be sites of arrhythmogenic foci requiring ablation within the sinuses.

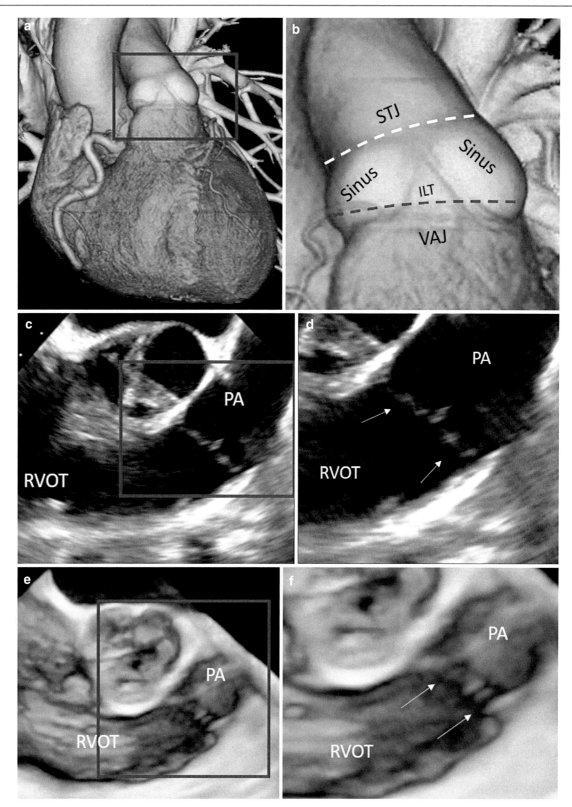

Fig. 6.21 (**a**) CT image volume-rendering format. The area within the red box is magnified in (**b**). The magnified image clearly shows the sinu-tubular junction (STJ), marked by a white dotted line, the interleaf-let triangle (ILT), and the ventriculo-arterial junction (VAJ) marked with a red dotted line. (**c**) 2D transesophageal echocardiography in long-axis view of the right ventricular outflow tract (RVOT). The area within the red box is magnified in (**d**). Images clearly show the pulmo-nary leaflets (*arrows*). (**e**) Same images as in (**c**) in 3D format. The area within the red box is magnified in (**f**). *Arrows* indicate pulmonary leaf-lets. *PA* pulmonary artery

Suggested Reading

Epstein FH. MRI of left ventricular function. J Nucl Cardiol. 2007;14(5):729–44.

Fernandez-Teran MA, Hrule JM. Myocardial fiber architecture of the human heart. Anat Rec. 1982;204:137–47.

Ho SY. Anatomy and myoarchitecture of the left ventricular wall in normal and in disease. Eur J Echocardiogr. 2009;10:i3–7.

Ho SY, Nihoyannopoulos P. Anatomy, echocardiography, and normal right ventricular dimensions. Heart. 2006;92(Suppl I):i2–13.

Maffei E, Messalli G, Martini C, et al. Left and right ventricle assessment with cardiac CT: validation study vs. cardiac MR. Eur Radiol. 2012;22(5):1041–9.

Sheehan F, Redington A. The right ventricle: anatomy, physiology and clinical imaging. Heart. 2008;94:1510–5.

Stamm C, Anderson RH, Ho SY. Clinical anatomy of the normal pulmonary root compared with that in isolated pulmonary valve stenosis. J Am Coll Cardiol. 1998;31(6):1420–5.

The Coronary Arteries and Veins

7

Francesco F. Faletra, Marco Araco, Laura A. Leo,
Giovanni Pedrazzini, Tiziano Moccetti, Marco Moccetti,
Elena Pasotti, and Siew Yen Ho

Introduction

A deep understanding of human coronary arteries anatomy and spatial relationships between coronary vessels and surrounding myocardium helps to provide insights for interpreting invasive coronary angiography and recognizing potential ischemic territories. On the other hand, a sustained interest in the anatomy of the coronary veins system is due to the introduction of cardiac resynchronization therapy and to the development of new devices that are implanted in the coronary sinus with the aim to reduce functional mitral regurgitation. These topics will be covered extensively in this chapter. Finally, a brief paragraph on the histology of coronary arteries explains the relevant role of endothelium.

While in the previous chapters echocardiography, CT, and CMR have been used to illustrate cardiac anatomy, in this chapter the anatomy of coronary vessels is almost exclusively illustrated by CT and by a new "entry": invasive coronary angiography (ICA). Indeed, both echocardiography and CMR are not the most appropriate techniques for illustrating the anatomy of the coronary arteries. The reasons are explained in the following paragraphs.

The Marginal Role of Echocardiography and CMR in Visualizing Coronary Arteries

A huge amount of studies has indisputably documented the role of stress echocardiography in detecting myocardial ischemia caused by coronary artery disease (CAD).Conversely, very few studies have investigated the role of echocardiography in visualizing coronary arteries. These studies have shown that, using high frequency transthoracic and transesophageal transducers, short segments of coronary arteries can be visualized. However, because of its intrinsic tomographic nature, transecting vessels in long-axis view requires a vessel's straight course, which is often not the case for coronary arteries because they usually have tortuous paths. Moreover, a vessel with a diameter of less than 2 mm may scarcely be visualized due to the relatively low resolution of echocardiography. Thus, direct visualization of coronary arteries is not part of the routine echocardiographic examination.

In clinical practice cardiologists require CMR stress-rest myocardial perfusion (MP) and late gadolinium enhancement imaging (LGE) to assess myocardial ischemia and infarction. Less likely they require a direct visualization of coronary arteries. Yet, in experienced hands, CMR can visualize almost the entire coronary tree, and several studies have shown that this technique may achieve good accuracy when compared with ICA in distinguishing normal from diseased coronary arteries (especially when combined with MP and LGE). However, visualizing the entire coronary tree with CMR is a complicated procedure. Acquisition protocol, in fact, is rather complex and time-consuming (navigator-gated, electrocardiogram [ECG]-triggered, fat-saturated, inversion-recovery prepared segmented and 3D gradient-echo sequence) and a complete examination (including LGE)

F. F. Faletra (✉) · L. A. Leo
Non-invasive Cardiovascular Imaging Department, Fondazione Cardiocentro Ticino, Lugano, Switzerland
e-mail: Francesco.Faletra@cardiocentro.org; lauraanna.leo@cardiocentro.org

M. Araco · M. Moccetti
Interventional Cardiology Department, Fondazione Cardiocentro Ticino, Lugano, Switzerland
e-mail: marco.araco@cardiocentro.org; marco.moccetti@cardiocentro.org

G. Pedrazzini · T. Moccetti · E. Pasotti
Cardiology Department, Fondazione Cardiocentro Ticino, Lugano, Switzerland
e-mail: giovanni.pedrazzini@cardiocentro.org; tiziano.moccetti@cardiocentro.org; elena.pasotti@cardiocentro.org

S. Y. Ho
Royal Brompton Hospital, Sydney Street, London, UK
e-mail: yen.ho@imperial.ac.uk

© Springer Nature Switzerland AG 2020
F. F. Faletra et al. (eds.), *Atlas of Non-Invasive Imaging in Cardiac Anatomy*, https://doi.org/10.1007/978-3-030-35506-7_7

takes no less than 1 h. During coronary image acquisition, patients are asked to breath regularly to avoid deep breathing and shallow breathing (which is not always simple). Even when the examination is performed correctly, diagnostic quality of coronary images in individual segments may be unpredictably poor, due to persistence of motion artifacts. Finally, the spatial resolution of the system does not allow visualizing of secondary branches of the epicardial coronary arteries. Last but not least, there is limited availability of the use of CMR for this purpose. Thus, for many cardiologists the direct visualization of coronary arteries with CMR,

although possible, is considered a "boutique" modality. HASTE sequences, on the contrary, have been used routinely to rule-out abnormal origin of coronary arteries in those patients in whom it is preferable to avoid radiation exposure. In conclusion, like echocardiography, CMR is better tailored to assess functional than anatomical coronary disease, and consequently it does not appear to be the best method for illustrating the anatomy of coronary arteries (Fig. 7.1).

Because of the inconsistency in imaging coronary arteries by echocardiography and technical and practical difficulties in obtaining comprehensive images of the coronary tree with

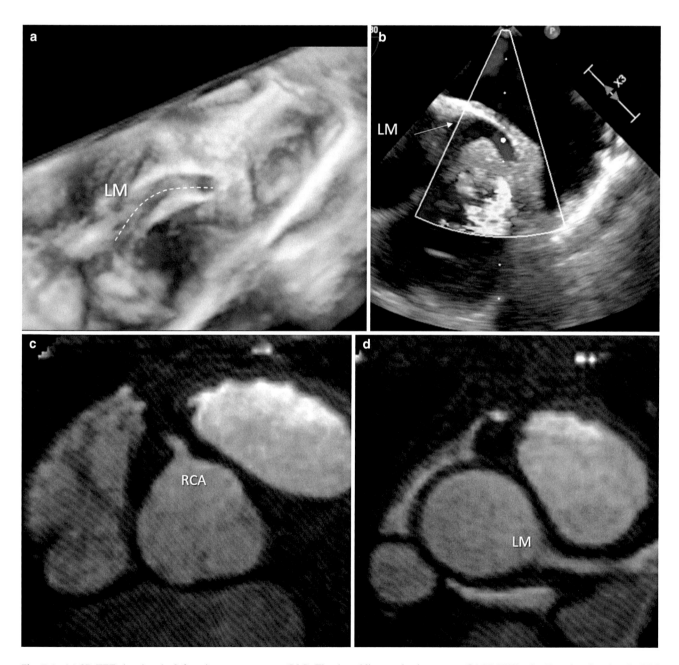

Fig. 7.1 (a) 3D TEE showing the left main coronary artery (LM). The dotted line marks the course. (b) 2D TEE color Doppler showing the LM flow (arrow). (c and d) HASTE acquisitions showing the origin of right coronary artery (RCA) and left main coronary artery (LM), respectively

CMR, in this chapter we describe the anatomy of coronary vessels using ICA, and the "noninvasive" coronary angiography (CTCA). It could be useful for readers to understand advantages and disadvantages of both techniques.

Advantages and Disadvantages of ICA

The first invasive selective coronary angiogram was reported in 1959 by Mason Sones, a pediatric cardiologist from the Cleveland Clinic. While performing an angiography of the aortic root, Sones wrongly manipulated the catheter, which accidentally entered in the right coronary artery. Before it was removed, a small amount of contrast agent opacified the right coronary artery. This became the world's first selective coronary angiography. A few years later, other pioneers such as Seldinger, Abrams, and Judkins introduced the transfemoral approach and more dedicated catheters. Over the decades, continuous technical advancements of fluoroscopic imaging systems, development of less toxic contrast agents, and new high-performance catheters and guide wires, have made ICA as it is today: a remarkably effective imaging technique for visualizing coronary arteries. Moreover, it remains the only method capable of assessing coronary vessels as small as 1 mm, collateral circulation, vasospasm and, to some extent, coronary perfusion (Fig. 7.2).

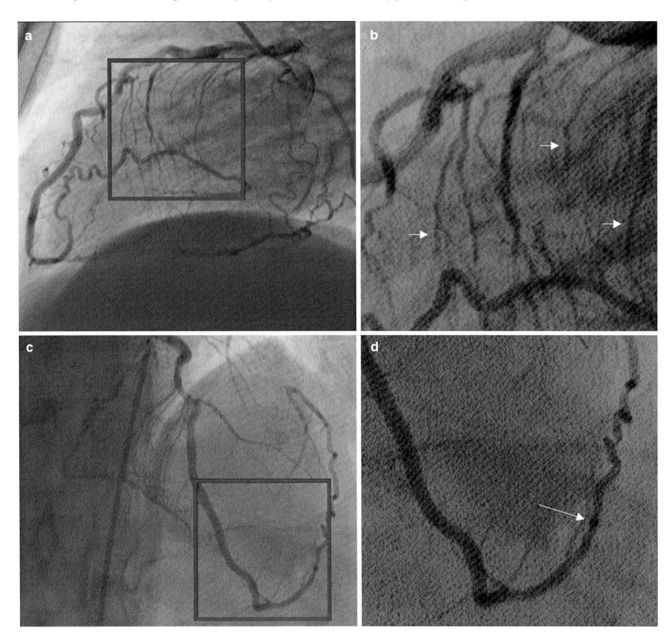

Fig. 7.2 Invasive coronary angiography (ICA). The areas in the red box of panels (**a**) and (**c**) are magnified in panels (**b**) and (**d**) respectively. Images show that the ICA can visualize very small coronary branches (arrows in panel **b**) and collateral vessels (arrow in panel **d**)

ICA has had an enormous impact on clinical cardiology, offering an optimal management of ischemic heart disease. Without ICA neither surgical nor percutaneous revascularization would have been possible. Currently, millions of ICA are performed worldwide annually.

ICA, however, has its own limitations:

(a) It is an "invasive" technique. As with any invasive procedure, there are specific patient-dependent and procedure-related complications that are inherent to the examination. Complications range widely from minor problems with short-term sequelae to life-threatening situations that may cause irreversible damage. Fortunately, life-threatening complications are very uncommon (mortality less than 0.08%), and in experienced hands the procedure can be successfully performed with relatively low risk even in the most critically ill patient. Complications of the vascular access site are the most common and the most significant contributors to morbidity of the procedure. Lower profile catheters and smaller sheaths, as well as more effective vascular closure devices and an increased use of radial access, have reduced the incidence of vascular complications. Today in high-volume cath-lab the total vascular complications (including large inguinal hematoma, pseudoaneurysm, retroperitoneal hemorrhage, and arteriovenous fistula) are less than 1%.

(b) ICA visualizes the "lumen" of the vessels. It does not visualize the coronary artery wall. Atheromatous plaques of coronary arteries grow not only into the lumen, narrowing it (phenomenon visible to ICA), but also into the arterial wall (the so-called "positive remodeling"), which is "invisible" to ICA. Consequently, the true extent of atheromatous plaques is usually underestimated.

(c) ICA could be considered a "three-dimensional luminogram" displayed in a two-dimensional format. Optimal visualization of the coronary tree therefore requires at least two "triple orthogonal views," i.e., projections orthogonal to each other and to the target vessel. To lay out the entire normal coronary tree, at least 4–6 projections for the left coronary artery and 2–4 for the right coronary artery are necessary (see below). Additional projections may be necessary to overcome vessel overlap, tortuosity, and foreshortening.

(d) It is worth remembering that ICA carries the risks related to radiation exposure and contrast administration. A typical adult diagnostic coronary angiogram is performed with an x-ray exposure of 5–10 mSv and administration of 50–70 cc of iodinated contrast. Hence to reduce the radiation exposure and the risk of kidney injury, cardiologists performing ICA should strive to obtain the minimum number of indispensable projections.

Advantages and Disadvantages of CTCA

The first commercial CT scanner was literally "invented and built" by Sir Godfrey Hounsfield in 1967 and installed at Atkinson Morley Hospital in Wimbledon, England, in 1971. The same year, a similar CT scanner was built by Allan MacLeod Cormack at the Tufts University of Boston. In 1979, Hounsfield and Cormack won the Nobel Prize in Medicine.

While CT technology was ready in early 1980s to generate diagnostic images for immobile body organs, this was not yet achievable for the heart and, in particular, for coronary arteries. Indeed, cardiac motion and spatial resolution were the two main technical problems in obtaining diagnostic images of coronary arteries with CT. The fast movement of coronary arteries during the cardiac cycle requires high temporal resolution to "freeze" coronary arteries and avoid "blurring" of images due to motion artifacts; on the other hand, a spatial resolution at least of 1 mm is necessary to visualize the lumen of epicardial coronary arteries with diameters ranging from 4 to 1.5 mm.

From the beginning of the twenty-first century, new technological developments such as the introduction of multi-slice CT scanners, specific ECG-gated algorithms for partial-scan image reconstruction, and gantry rotation times below 1 s, provided the prerequisite for obtaining the first diagnostic images of coronary arteries relatively free of motion artifacts. Within a few years, the technology evolved at an unimaginable speed relative to other imaging modalities. The main technological progresses that enabled diagnostic images of coronary arteries today were:

(a) Gantry rotation times below 300 ms, which allows temporal resolution below 150 ms, because only half a rotation is needed to acquire the data required for the image reconstruction;

(b) Detector arrays up to 320 detector rows (a 320 detector rows CT covers the entire heart volume in one gantry rotation and one heartbeat);

(c) Dual source CT with two tube-detector systems off-set 90° to each other mounted in the same gantry that allow further reduction of the temporal resolution at one half of the single tube-detector;

(d) New image reconstruction algorithms.

These technological developments have led to an astonishing improvement in imaging quality with a spatial resolution of 0.6 mm and temporal resolution as low as 80 ms.

Two major issues must be mentioned:

(a) **_Radiation exposure_**. The ICRP (International Commission on Radiological Protection) estimated that the chance of acquiring fatal radiogenic cancer in the adult population is approximately 0.005%/mSv. In other words, as with any other imaging examination that exposes the patient to ionizing radiation (including ICA as above-mentioned), CTCA results in an increased incidence of radiation-induced cancer in the long-term. Despite the awareness of radiation risk and despite the huge radiation exposure produced by the first-generation CT scanners, this problem was almost disregarded at the beginning, or at best was significantly under estimated by radiologists and cardiologists (with a few exceptions). Some cardiologists justified the need of CTCA with the belief that the benefits of being aware of the coronary status of a given patient outweighs the harmful effects of high radiation exposure; whereas others simply do not consider this factor when requesting CTCA examinations. After a few years, however, the general awareness that the radiation issue became relevant not only for the individual patient but also for the community (because small individual risks multiplied by millions of examinations had become a significant population risk) led manufacturers to undertake new strategies to reduce radiation exposure as much as possible without compromising image quality. In many respects they succeeded. Today, in fact, the modern CT scan machines allow clear and accurate diagnostic images to be obtained with radiation dose exposure constantly in a range of 2–5 mSv (though in selected cases radiation exposure may be less than 1 mSv), which is significantly less than for ICA. We are convinced that the inherent risk of radiation-induced fatal malignancy, though very low and over the long-term, should always be weighed against the risks of a CAD remaining undetected. Finally, we completely agree with the statement recently provided by European Society of Cardiology: "A smart physician cannot be afraid of the essential and often life-saving use of medical radiation, but must be very afraid of radiation unawareness."

(b) *Appropriateness*. The rapid growth and dissemination of CTCA has raised concerns regarding its overuse in the clinical setting. Indeed, while an appropriate use should likely improve patient clinical outcomes, inappropriate use of CTCA may be potentially harmful to patients and may also generate unwarranted costs to the health care system. Herein we limit to reporting the definition of appropriateness according to guidelines: "An appropriate imaging study is one in which the expected incremental information, combined with clinical judgment, exceeds the expected negative consequences by a sufficiently wide margin for a specific indication that the procedure is generally considered acceptable care and a reasonable approach for the indication."

From an anatomic point of view, coronary arteries are exquisitely illustrated by using CT three-dimensional volume rendering, which shows images of epicardial arteries that closely resemble actual gross anatomy. This 3D volume rendering algorithm uses a threshold for displaying structures that are above a certain CT attenuation, generally showing the contrast-enhanced blood pool. Thus, cardiac chambers, great vessels, and coronary arteries filled with contrasted blood are well visualized. The myocardium of left and right ventricles is, at least partially, opacified because the contrast perfuses through small vessels and capillaries. As a result, this algorithm is able to reconstruct amazing pictures of epicardial coronary arteries running over the right and left ventricular cavities (Fig. 7.3).

Other qualities make CTCA an ideal anatomy-teaching tool for coronary arteries. The abilities to "fly around," that is, to rotate the 3D data set to obtain a virtually countless number of perspectives, and "to zoom in" on specific areas, allow a precise understanding of the distribution of the main epicardial arteries and their branches (Figs. 7.3 and 7.4). The ability to delete cardiac structures that cover segments of coronary arteries makes CTCA similar to cadaveric dissection. Figure 7.4 shows that the mid-segment of the right coronary artery running on the atrio-ventricular groove, and usually covered by the overlapping atrial cavity, can be made visible by cropping the right atrial cavity.

The ability to make the myocardium transparent, while maintaining the coronary vessels opacified, allows clear images of coronary distribution to be obtained (Fig. 7.5).

Finally, single vessels may be visualized using multiplanar reconstruction image, an algorithm which projects the entire course of a vessel in a single plane, despite the fact that a tortuous vessel may travel through many planes. This modality is usually used to detect coronary stenosis, and not for illustrating anatomical course of the vessels, since the anatomical relationships with surrounding myocardium are distorted (Fig. 7.6). Thus, for the purpose of this chapter we explicitly use the volume rendering modality.

However, it should be said that CTCA does not perform equally well in all patients. A stable, low heart rate (65–70 bpm) is required at the time of the examination because, even with the latest generation of scanner machines, motion artifacts can occur. Oral or intravenous β-blockers should be administered before the study to maintain a regular heart rate at rest and to reduce heart rate variability during the scan. Because image quality is often suboptimal in patients with irregular heart rates, scanning patients during atrial fibrillation should be avoided. Similarly, aborting a scan is a reasonable option if frequent ventricular ectopyis present. Breathing during the scan is another issue because it significantly compromises image quality and produces segments of coronary arteries that cannot be evaluated. If the patient cannot hold the breath for 5–10 s he or she should not be scanned. Intravenous iodinated contrast material is needed to visualize the coronary arteries; thus, the procedure is contraindicated

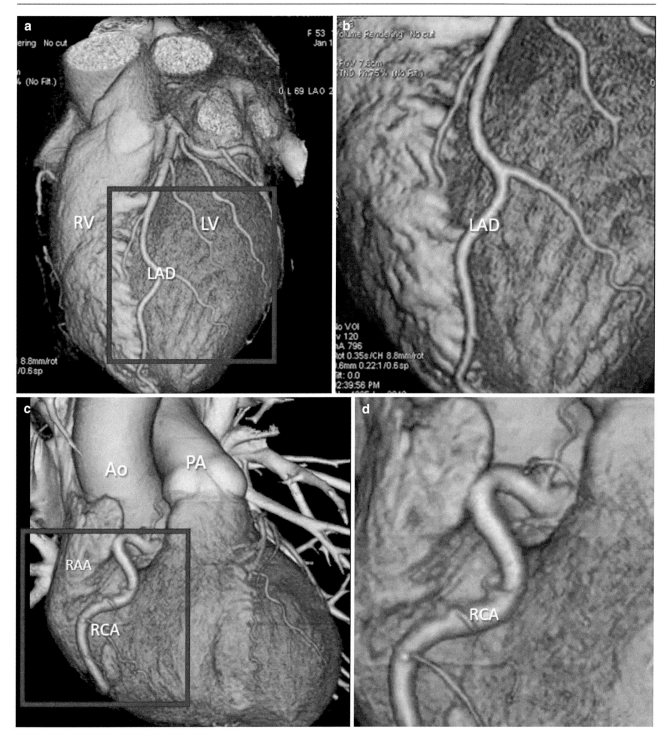

Fig. 7.3 (a and c) CT volume-rendering modality showing the right (RV) and left (LV) ventricles from a left oblique (a) and from an anterior (c) perspective respectively. The areas in the red boxes are magnified in panels (b) and (d). The left anterior descending artery (LAD) and the right coro-nary artery (RCA) are beautifully visualized. The right ventricle (RV) and the left ventricle (LV) are partially visualized because the contrast through small vessels and capillaries opacified the inner layers of myocardium (see text). *Ao* Aorta, *PA* pulmonary artery, *RAA* right atrial appendage

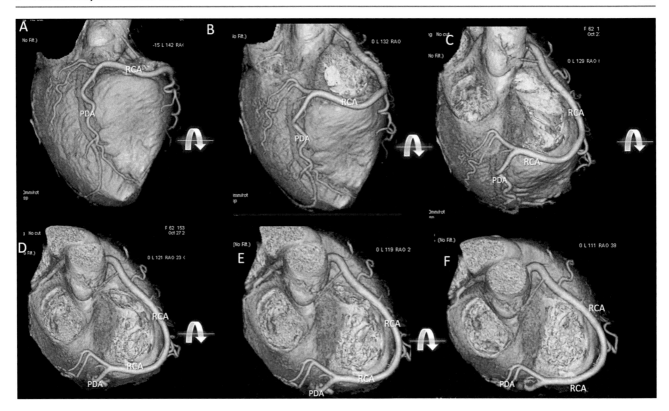

Fig. 7.4 (**A–F**) CT volume-rendering modality. The atrioventricular course of the right coronary artery (RCA) is made visible by deleting the atrial cavities and rotating the volume data set up-to-down around x-axis (curved arrow)

in some subjects with severe contrast material allergy. Subjects with a history of mild contrast material allergy should be premedicated with steroids and antihistamines before the scan. Similarly, the CTCA should be avoided in patients with high serum creatinine levels (glomerular filtration rate < 45 mL/min). Finally, in patients with body mass index of >40 kg/m², CTCA should be avoided, since diagnostic images are obtained at expense of a significant increase of radiation dose.

Anatomy of Coronary Artery

The term *coronary arteries and veins* derives from the Latin word *corona/coronaries*, which means *crown*. Indeed, the epicardial vessels running on the surface of the heart form two crowns around the heart. The first crown follows the anterior and posterior interventricular grooves and comprises the left descending artery (LDA), which runs on the anterior interventricular groove, and the right posterior descending artery (PDA), which travels on the posterior interventricular groove. The second crown follows the atrio-ventricular groove, and it is formed by the right coronary artery (RCA) and by the left circumflex artery (Cx) (Fig. 7.7).

From a didactic point of view the coronary arteries can be divided into three segments; two of them, i.e., left anterior descending (LAD) and left circumflex arteries (LCx), usually take their origin from the left main coronary artery (LM), which arises from the left coronary sinus of the aorta. The third segment the right coronary artery (RCA) arises from right coronary sinus (Fig. 7.8).

The Left Coronary Artery

The left coronary artery originates from the left coronary sinuses, usually from a single ostium. The proximal part is called left main coronary artery (LM). It has an initial diameter of 4–5 mm and runs leftward within the transverse pericardial sinus beyond the back of the pulmonary infundinulum/pulmonary trunk for 5–15 mm; then it divides into two main vessels: the circumflex artery (LCx) and the left descending coronary artery (LAD). In some cases, a third vessel (the intermediate branch) originates from the angle between LAD and LCx, creating a trifurcation of LM. Given the oblique orientation of the heart, the long axis of LM is usually parallel to the horizontal plane of the thorax (Fig. 7.9).

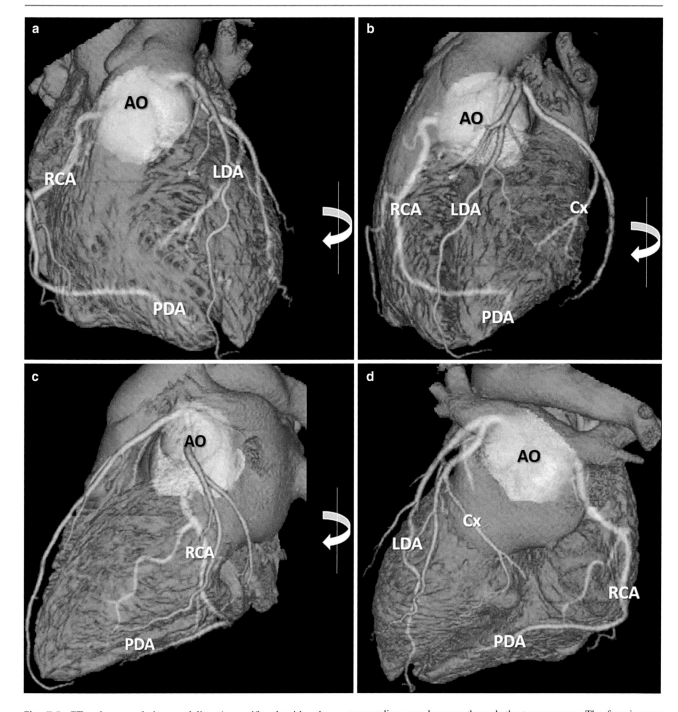

Fig. 7.5 CT volume-rendering modality. A specific algorithm has made the myocardium transparent, leaving the aortic root (AO) and the coronary tree opaque. Thus, coronary arteries running posteriorly to the myocardium can be seen through the transparency. The four images (**a–d**) have been rotated left-to-right around the y-axis (curved arrows) to show the coronary tree from different perspectives

The Left Anterior Descending Artery (LAD)

Continuing directly from the LM that emerges to the left of the pulmonary artery, the LAD turns inferiorly to enter the interventricular groove and runs to the apex of the heart. Along its pathway the LAD is surrounded by epicardial fat. In some instances, the vessel continues around the apex

ascending into the posterior interventricular groove to some extent. The importance of the LAD is that it serves a large amount of myocardium. Indeed, the LAD gives raise to three types of branches:

- *The diagonal branches*, of which there may be up to six, which course leftwards supplying the antero-lateral wall

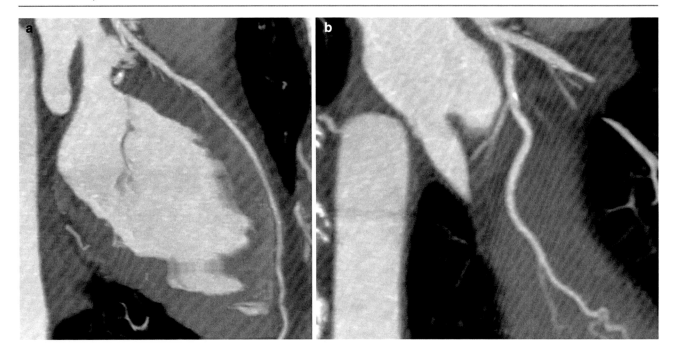

Fig. 7.6 CT multiplanar reconstruction of LAD (**a**) and left circumflex artery (LCx) (**b**). Although the coronary arteries have a tortuous course passing through many planes, this algorithm projects the entire course of the coronary vessel in a single plane. Of course, the anatomical relationships between cardiac chambers are distorted

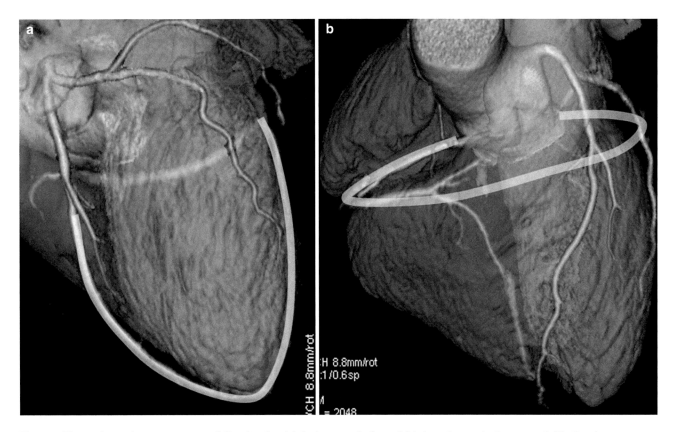

Fig. 7.7 Electronic cast in transparency modality showing (**a**) the interventricular and (**b**) the atrio-ventricular crowns (white lines)

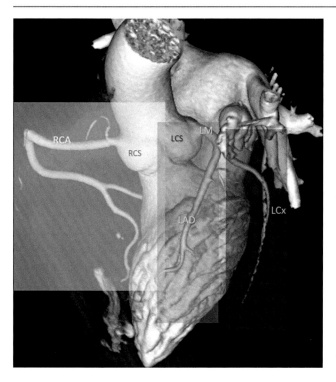

Fig. 7.8 CT electronic cast showing the classic subdivision of coronary arteries in three segments. Two of them, the left anterior descending (LAD) and left circumflex artery (LCx), usually originate from the left main coronary artery (LM), which arises from the left coronary sinus (LCS) of the aorta. The third segment, the right coronary artery (RCA), arises from right coronary sinus (RCS). The yellow box includes the RCA, while the blue and red boxes include the LAD and LCx, respectively

of the left ventricle. Occasionally, the first diagonal branch may be as large as the LAD. In such a case some septal branches may take their origin from this "twin LAD" (Fig. 7.10).

- *The septal branches* run perpendicular to the LAD and supply the interventricular septum. The first and second septal branches are usually the largest. Septal branches are well visible with ICA, and less visible with CTCA due to their small sizes. These small coronary branches have surged to clinical attention as targets for one of the treatments of patients with hypertrophic cardiomyopathy (HCM) and intraventricular obstruction. In HCM, intraventricular obstruction is caused by a very thick basal part of interventricular septum that protrudes into the left ventricular outflow tract associated with an anterior systolic displacement of the tip of the mitral valve toward the septum. Medical therapy with beta-blockers, calcium antagonists, and disopyramide is the first-line treatment to reduce symptoms and improve quality of life. For patients with drug-refractory symptoms and persistent significant outflow obstruction, surgical myectomy has been the treatment of choice. The proce-

dure removes part of the protruding septal myocardium via a transaortic approach and is associated with symptom improvement and reduction in cardiovascular mortality. An alternative to surgical myectomy is percutaneous treatment based on injection of a small amount of alcohol into one of the septal branches. The procedure causes a localized necrosis of the septal bulge. Intraprocedural contrast echocardiography is used as a guide to select the correct septal branch that supplies the septal area to be treated. The treatment is generally effective, leading to a slowly progressive reduction of intraventricular gradient (as long as scar substitutes the necrotic area) and improvement of symptoms. The septal lesion caused by the procedure closely resemble that produced by surgical myectomy. The most dreaded complication remains the development of atrio-ventricular block. This is not surprising because the first septal branch supplies blood to the right bundle branch, and in many cases also supplies the atrio-ventricular conduction bundle (Fig. 7.11).

- Finally, *the right ventricular branches*, are small arteries that run rightward from the LAD supplying the anterior-lateral wall of the right ventricle.

The Left Circumflex Artery (LCx)

In a normal morphological aspect, the LCx arises from the LM at a right angle to the LAD, creating a bifurcation. After its origin the LCx travels just inferior to left atrial appendage. This anatomical relationship should be taken into account during the occlusion of the appendage with a device, since the radial forces of the device could damage the artery (Fig. 7.12).

The vessel goes into the atrio-ventricular groove, surrounded by abundant epicardial fat, before descending the obtuse margin of the left ventricle as the marginal branch. The remaining course of LCx is extremely variable. In hearts with right coronary dominance the atrioventricular segment of the LCx may be short, ending in a marginal branch that is often larger and longer than the LCx itself. In left-dominant systems the LCx continues around the left atrioventricular groove to reach the crux and gives rise to the posterior descending artery. At the crux, one of its branches supplies the atrio-ventricular node. In a balanced dominance, the primary branches of LCx are the marginal branches (two or three in number) which supply the lateral wall of the left ventricle. The first marginal branch is usually the largest and the longest. In almost 30% of hearts, a small vessel arising from the LCx and running upward into the left atrium supplies the sinus node (Fig. 7.13).

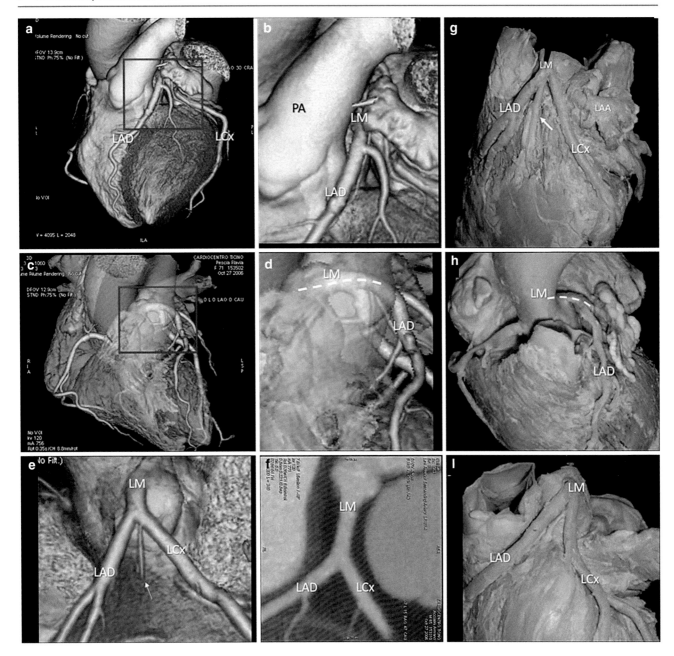

Fig. 7.9 (**a**) CT volume-rendering modality. The area in the red box is magnified in panel (**b**). The images show the course of the left main coronary artery (LM) posterior to the pulmonary artery (PA). (**c**) CT volume-rendering modality with transparency of the right (RV) and left (LV) ventricles. The area in the red box is magnified in panel (**d**). The LM is posterior to the PA and its long axis is parallel to the horizontal plane of the thorax (dotted line). (**e** and **f**) Volume-rendering CT and multiplanar reconstruction format showing the LM dividing in the left anterior descending artery (LAD) and into the left circumflex artery (LCX). The arrow points to a small intermediate branch. (**g–i**) The corresponding anatomical specimens. In panel (**g**) the arrow points at the intermediate branch

The Right Coronary Artery (RCA)

The RCA arises from the right coronary sinus. The initial part of RCA travels through the fatty tissues occupying the space between the right atrial appendage and the right outflow tract (Fig. 7.14).

In its first portion the RCA gives rise to a small artery supplying the right ventricular infundibulum (conus artery). From this portion the first atrial branch is the sinus node artery in nearly 70% of cases. It ascends in the interatrial groove to reach the sinus node located at the antero-lateral junction between the superior vena cava and the right atrium. After a short initial course, the RCA runs into the right atrio-ventricular groove surrounded by abundant epicardial fat. Of note is the anatomical relationship of RCA with the hinge-line of mural leaflet of tricuspid valve, the so-called tricuspid annulus (TA). Indeed, the RCA runs very close to the TA (Fig. 7.15).

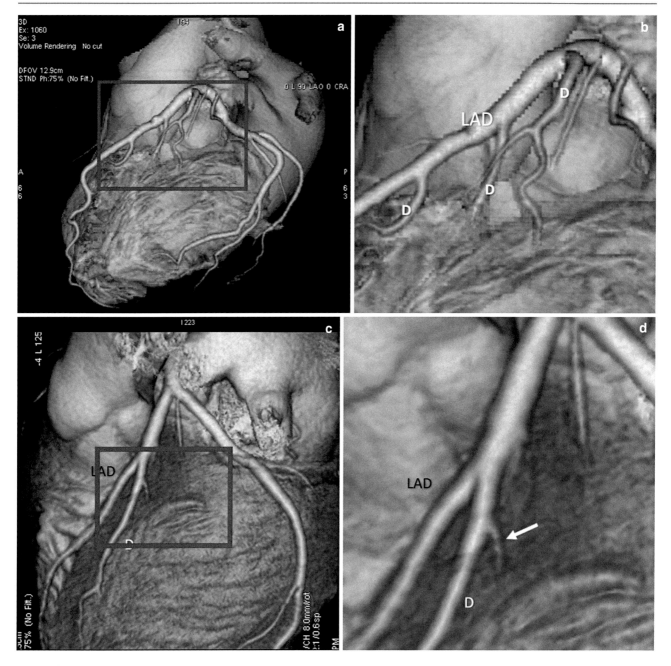

Fig. 7.10 (**a**) CT volume-rendering with transparency in lateral perspective. The area in the red box is magnified in panel (**b**). Image shows three diagonal branches (D) arising from the left anterior descending artery (LAD). (**c**) Volume-rendering format showing a large diagonal.

The area in the red box is magnified in panel (**d**). In the magnified image a very thin septal branch takes origin from a large diagonal (arrow)

Since the TA is frequently the target for surgical or percutaneous implant of a prosthetic ring, the precise position in each segment between the RCA and TA is crucial information for both cardiac surgeons and interventional cardiologists (see also Chap. 3).

The right marginal branches supply the anterior free wall of the RV. Distally the RCA divides into the posterior descending coronary artery (PDA) and posterior left ventricular branches: the PDA arises from the right coronary artery in 70–80% of cases (right dominance) and travels along the posterior interventricular groove surrounded by epicardial fat. The PDA supplies septal perforator branches into the posterior (inferior) half of the interventricular septum (Fig. 7.16).

At the crux, the dominant RCA makes a U-bend from which a small but important vessel, the atrio-ventricular node artery, arises to penetrate the fat-filled posterior (inferior) pyramidal space to reach the node. Finally, before

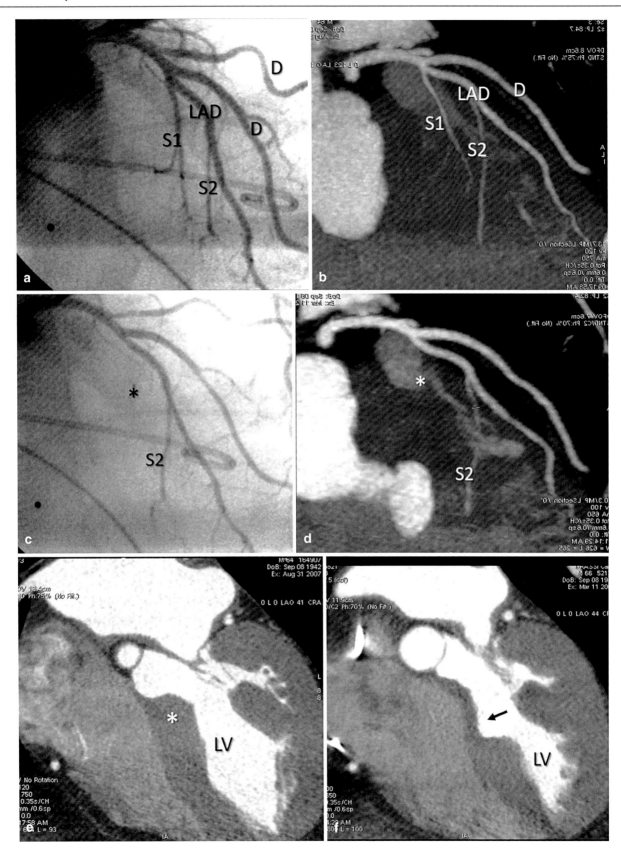

Fig. 7.11 (a) ICA and (b) CTCA showing two septal branches (S1, S2) arising from the left descending coronary artery (LAD). (c and d) Same images of panel (a) and (b) after alcohol ablation of the S1. The vessel is no longer visible (asterisk). (e) CT showing the left ventricle and the septal bulge (asterisk) before the procedure and (f) after the procedure. The reduction of the septal bulge is evident (arrow). D Diagonal branches

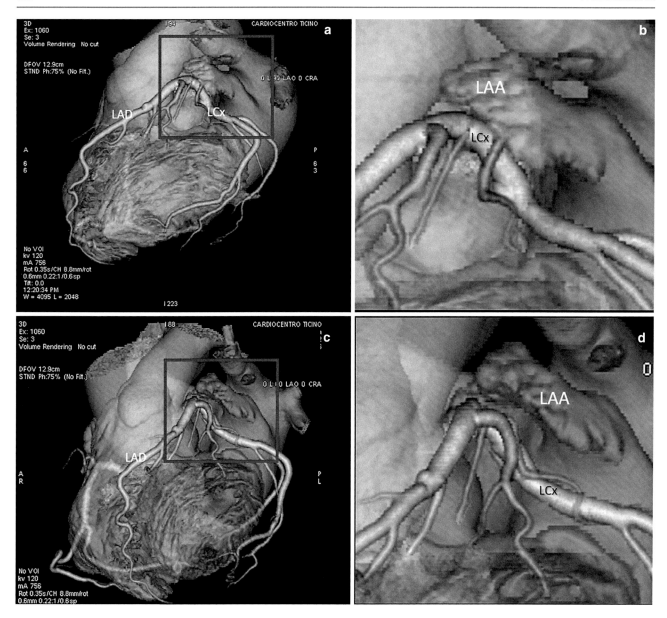

Fig. 7.12 (**a** and **c**) CT volume-rendering modality (transparency mode) from two slightly different lateral perspectives. The left descending coronary artery (LAD) and the left circumflex artery (LCx) are very well depicted. The areas in red boxes are magnified in panel (**b**) and (**d**) respectively. It is clearly visible as the LCx passes just under the left atrial appendage (LAA)

ending, the RCA sends a variable number of posterior lateral branches that supply the posterior-inferior (diaphragmatic) wall of the left ventricle and the posterior medial papillary muscle of the mitral valve.

Epicardial Adipose Tissue

The epicardial adipose tissue (EAT) that surrounds the epicardial coronary arteries and their branches is a mix of adipocytes and inflammatory, stromal, and immune cells secreting bioactive molecules, wrapped up by a network of fine connective fibers and nourished by a rich microcirculation. This heterogeneous composition reveals that the EAT is a truly biologically active organ that has a protective and, at the same time, harmful effect on epicardial coronary arteries. Anatomists noted the absence of a connective lamina layer separating EAT from the coronary vessels. In other words, the EAT is in direct contact with the adventitia of coronary arteries. It is logical, therefore, to postulate that EAT may interact locally with the coronary arteries through paracrine secretions of pro-inflammatory and pro-atherogenic molecules. Indeed, there is substantial evidence demonstrating the association between EAT and coronary atherosclerosis. On

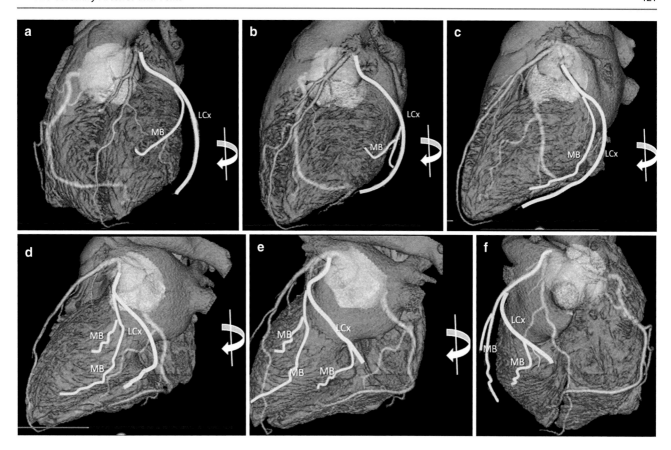

Fig. 7.13 (**a–f**) CT volume-rendering (transparency mode) showing in the balanced dominance, the course of circumflex artery (LCx) and marginal branches (MB) in different perspectives (yellow line) obtained rotating the 3D data set right-to-left around the Y axis (curved arrow)

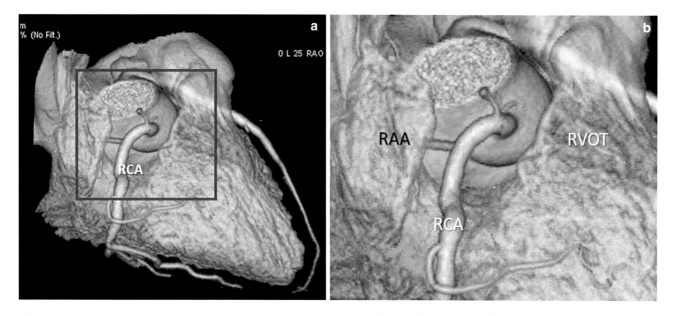

Fig. 7.14 (**a**) CT volume-rendering modality (transparency mode) showing the proximal and mid segments of the right coronary artery (RCA). The area in the red box is magnified in panel (**b**). The figure shows the proximal segment of the RCA between the right atrial appendage (RAA) and the right ventricular outflow tract (RVOT)

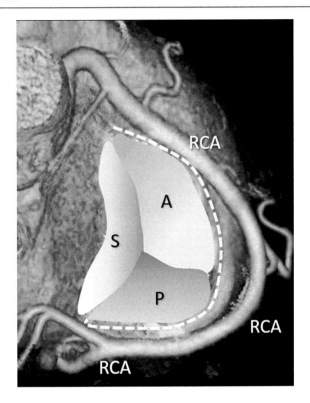

Fig. 7.15 CT volume-rendering format. The right atrium has been removed to visualize the atrioventricular course of the right coronary artery (RCA) and its anatomical relationship with the mural segment of tricuspid annulus (curved white dotted line). Superimposed is a depiction of the tricuspid leaflets: septal (S), anterior (A) and posterior (P)

the other hand, EAT also produces protective, anti-inflammatory and antiatherogenic adipokines. Moreover, surrounding the major coronary arteries, EAT provides a mechanical protection of the coronary arteries, buffering them against the torsion induced by the arterial pulse wave and cardiac contraction. The EAT and its relationship with the coronary arteries can be beautifully visualized by CMR and CT (Fig. 7.17).

Angiographic Projections of Coronary Arteries

Many textbooks and atlases have extensively described and illustrated x-ray projections for obtaining optimal views of coronary arteries. Yet cardiologists-in-training and experienced general cardiologists are quite unfamiliar with projections of ICA. The trickies tissue is to understand how the heart and coronary arteries move when changing projections.

The *theory* is simple: The catheterization laboratory is set with the x-ray source located underneath the patient and the image intensifier (or flat panel detector) above, moving in opposite directions around the patient in order to produce the angiographic projections. The direction of the flat panel determines any given angiographic view. In antero-posterior (AP) projection the flat panel is above the patient; in right

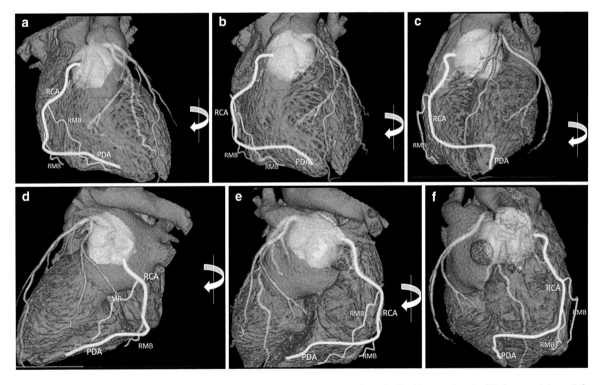

Fig. 7.16 (a–f) CT volume-rendering (transparency mode) showing the course (yellow line) of right coronary artery (RCA), posterior descending artery (PDA), and right marginal branches (RMB) in differ-ent perspectives obtained by rotating the 3D data set right-to-left around the Y axis (curved arrow)

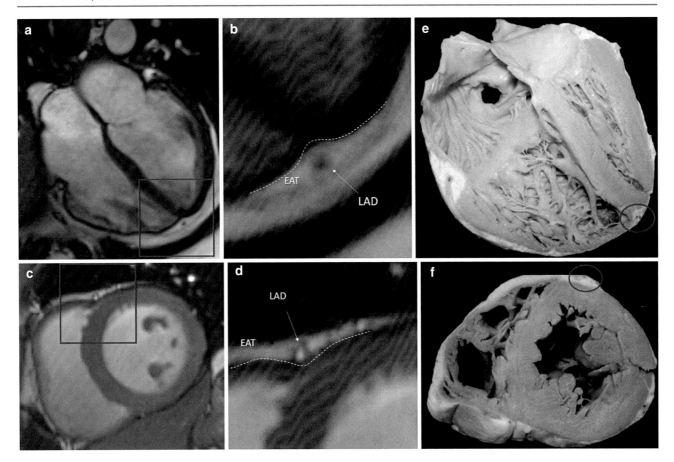

Fig. 7.17 (**a**) CMR in four-chamber view. The area in the red box is magnified in panel (**b**). The left descending coronary artery (LAD), near the apex (arrow), is surrounded by the epicardial adipose tissue (EAT). (**c**) CMR short-axis view. The area in the red box is magnified in panel (**d**). The LAD (arrow) runs in the interventricular groove (dotted line) surrounded by EAT. (**e**, **f**) The corresponding anatomic specimens. The red circles point at LAD near the apex (panel **e**) and at mid-ventricle (panel **f**)

anterior oblique (RAO) projection the flat panel moves to the right of the patient; and in left anterior oblique (LAO) projection the flat panel moves to the left. In cranial (CRA) views the flat panel is tilted toward the head of the patient, and in caudal (CAU) views it is tilted toward the feet. Furthermore, caudal projections are in general better suited for proximal segment visualization, while cranial projections are better for mid- and distal segments (Fig. 7.18).

The *practice* is *not* simple: One of the major difficulties arises from the fact that each individual's coronary arteries are unique and follow no common pathway. The distribution of coronary arteries and their branches, as well as size and length, are extremely variable. Moreover, CTCA volume-rendering modality provides pictures of coronary arteries along with the cast of heart cavities, which certainly helps in recognizing single vessel; ICA, however, does not provide this.

Today a comprehensive angiographic visualization of coronaries usually requires five or six for the left and two or three for the right coronary artery. But supplemental views are necessary when the study is inconclusive, or to define better intermediate coronary narrowing, or to avoid overlap and foreshortening or, finally, to choose the best angiographic view for PTCA. Figures 7.19, 7.20, and 7.21 offer a summary of the most frequent angiographic projections used to visualize the coronary arteries to familiarize beginners with this tough topic.

Coronary Distribution and Myocardium Segments

Obstruction or occlusion of a given coronary artery reduces or interrupts perfusion on downstream myocardium. The absence of blood supply causes a cascade of events that eventually leads to wall motion abnormality (WMA). There are different physio-pathological scenarios. WMA may be due either to stunned myocardium (which is a condition of "rescued" myocardium that exhibits a post-ischemic dysfunction), or to "hibernating" myocardium (which is a condition of "chronically" ischemic myocardium supplied by narrow coronary arteries). In both these conditions the myo-

Fig. 7.18 Scheme of various
X-ray projections (see text)

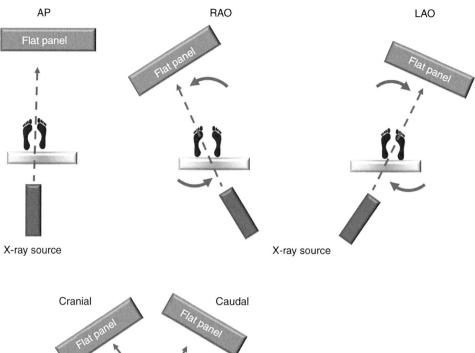

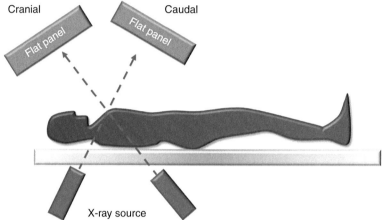

cardium is still viable, and WMA usually recovers spontane-
ously (in stunned myocardium), or after reperfusion (in
hibernating myocardium). Prolonged ischemia ultimately
causes an irreversible damage of the myocardium with cell
death and myocardial infarction.

With advent of 2D echocardiography in the 1960s, WMA
was graded as (1) *hypokinesis*, which consists in a reduction
of wall thickening and wall motion toward the center of the
ventricle; (2) *akinesis*, which consists in an absence of wall
thickening, though "passive" wall motion may persist
because the diseased myocardium may be tethered by the
normal contraction of adjacent segments; and (3) *dyskinesis*,
which consists of absence of wall thickening and "paradoxi-
cal" wall motion in which the diseased myocardial segments
are pushed away from the center of the ventricle. With the
advent of PTCA and CMR, another physio-pathological concept has become popular: the "myocardium area at risk,"
which is the area of myocardium that is threatened during an
acute occlusion of a coronary artery and can be rescued
(totally or partially) by an immediate reperfusion.

Although, as mentioned above, the coronary circulation is
extremely variable, some general rules can be made about
segmentation of LV myocardium and assignment of each segment to a given coronary territory, though it is easily comprehensible that some segments can be supplied by more than
one coronary artery or by different arteries due to variability
of coronary distribution. The left ventricle can be divided into
16 or 17 segments. This segmentation is well known by imagers who may accurately predict the diseased coronary artery
based on WMA. Briefly, the anterior half of interventricular
septum (IVS) is perfused by the septal branches, while the
anterior free wall of the left ventricle is perfused by the diagonal branches of the LAD. The lateral free wall is perfused by
the LCx. In the left-dominant circulation, the LCx also supplies the posterior/inferior free wall and the posterior half of
the interventricular septum (IVS) through the PDA. In the
right-dominant pattern, the posterior half of IVS is perfused
by the RCA, which also supplies the anterior, lateral, and posterior aspects of the right myocardium as well as the poste-
rior/inferior free wall of the left myocardium. The cardiac

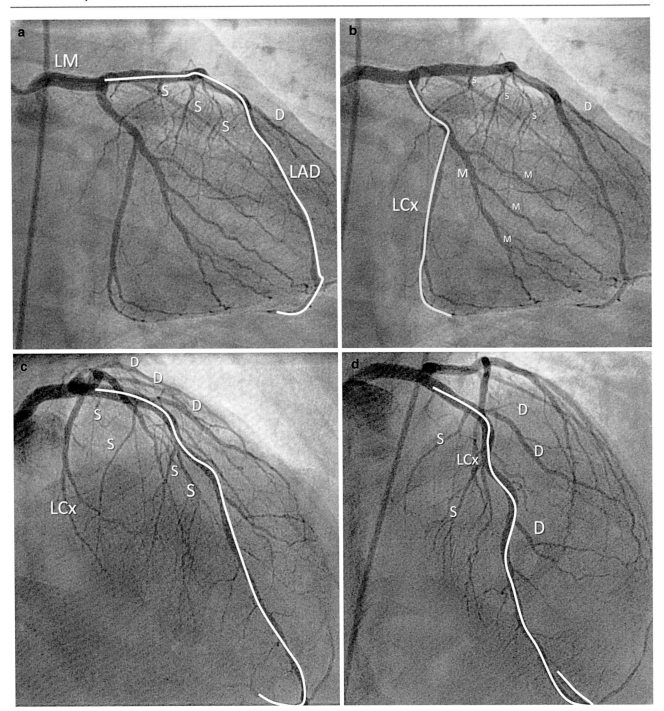

Fig. 7.19 Angiography of the left coronary artery in anterior-posterior projection (AP). In panel (**a**) the left main (LM) is visualized in its entire length (red line) while the white line marks the course of the proximal and mid left descending coronary artery (LAD) with diagonal (D) and septal (S) branches. In panel (**b**) the yellow line marks the course of the left circumflex artery with marginal branches (M). In panel (**c**) the right anterior oblique (RAO) cranial view and in panel (**d**) the AP cranial view, allow visualizing of the mid and distal LAD (white line) and the origin of its branches: diagonal branches (D), running to the right of the screen, and septal branches (S), downward and toward the left. The proximal LAD is often overlapped by the proximal left circumflex artery (LCx)

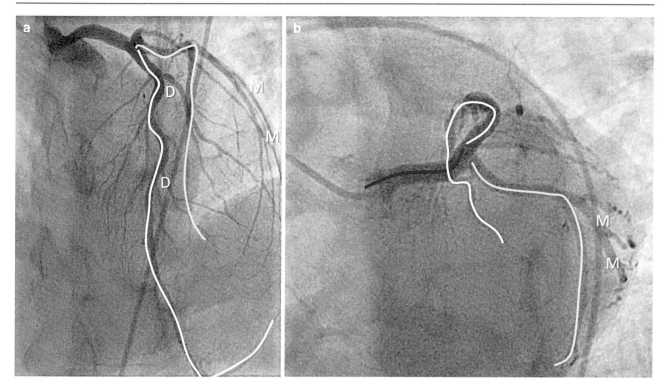

Fig. 7.20 In panel (a), the LAO cranial view shows the ostium of the left main coronary artery, the bifurcation into the proximal LAD and LCx, the LAD (white line) with the origin of the diagonal branches (D) and the LCx (yellow line) with marginal branches (M). In panel (b), LAO caudal view, also called spider, allows visualizing the left main (red line) and its bifurcation into the LAD (white line) and proximal and mid LCx (yellow line) with its marginal branches (M). Mid and distal segments of LAD are foreshortened

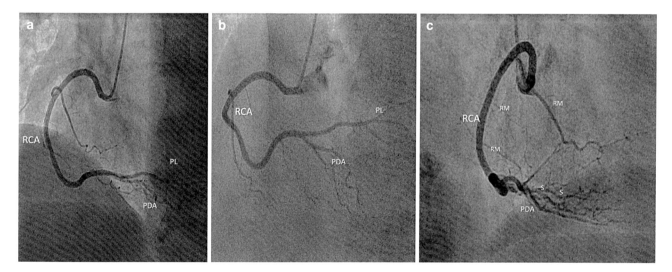

Fig. 7.21 In panel (a) the right coronary artery (RCA) is seen in LAO view. This view allows visualization of the proximal and mid RCA. The bifurcation of the distal RCA into posterior descending artery (PDA) and posterior-lateral branches (PL) is not well visualized and PDA and PL are foreshortened. In panel (b), cranial tilting of LAO allows better visualization of the PDA and PL; the mid RCA, however, is foreshortened. In the panel (c) the RAO projection shows the mid segment of the RCA with the origin of the right marginal branches and PDA, with septal branches running upward. Posterior-lateral branches are often overlapped. Finally, this is the best projection to visualize the bridging collaterals toward the LAD in case of LAD chronic total occlusion

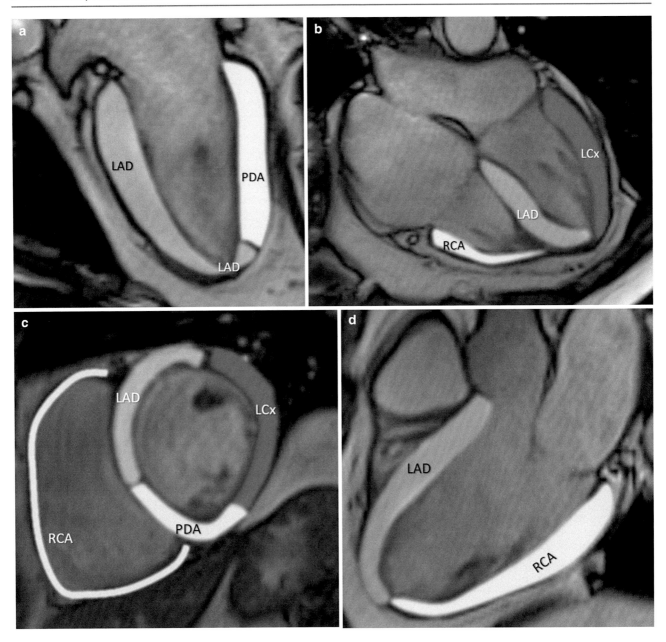

Fig. 7.22 A simplified collage of CMR images showing the most likely coronary distribution in a balanced coronary anatomy in (**a**) two-chamber view, (**b**) four-chamber view, (**c**) short-axis and (**d**) long axis views. *LAD* Left anterior descending artery, *RCA* Right coronary artery, *LCx* left circumflex artery, *PDA* posterior descending artery

apex is perfused by the LAD, which also supplies the apical third of the posterior wall when the LAD wraps around the apex. Figure 7.22 shows a simplified distribution of coronary territory in a balanced coronary anatomy.

The Microanatomy of Coronary Arteries

Like all arteries, the basic microstructure of the coronary artery comprises three distinct concentric layers termed intima, media, and adventitia. The *intima* consists of a lining layer of endothelial cell (endothelium) and a subendothelial layer of loose connective tissue with sparse connective and elastic fibers. The *endothelium* provides a smooth and selective barrier between the circulating blood and the other wall layers. The endothelial cells are orientated longitudinally relative to the long axis of the vessel. However, considering the endothelium as a simple barrier modulating diffusion of nutritional substances is reductive. Indeed, the endothelium is an *active organ* that has a number of metabolic and endocrine functions (considering all the arteries, the endothelium is one of the largest organs that interacts with nearly every other organ of the body). It is surprising, in fact, that a single monolayer of cells may have so many functions:

(a) Maintenance of hemostasis with a delicate equilibrium between antithrombotic and prothrombotic agents;
(b) Maintenance of an optimal permeability while at the same time acting as strong barrier to toxic materials;
(c) Control of angiogenesis;
(d) Maintenance of optimal vascular tone by modulating both vasoconstriction and vasodilation. This delicate modulation of coronary motricity permits an adequate end-organ perfusion. The control of local vascular tone is mediated principally by nitric oxide (NO), although other factors such as prostacyclin and endothelium-dependent hyperpolarization factor play an important role.

Thus, it is not surprising that endothelial dysfunction may produce a cascade of events leading to structural damage of arterial wall with smooth muscle cells proliferation, atherosclerotic plaque formation, and ultimately myocardial ischemia. In other words, atherosclerosis starts as a disease of the endothelium.

The intima is separated from the media layer by the internal elastic membrane, which is a fenestrated sheet of elastic tissue.

The *media* consists of multiple layers of smooth muscle cells surrounded by a mesh of connective and elastic fibers, wrapped up in a loose matrix of proteoglycans. It is interesting to note that the epicardial coronary arteries contain less elastic tissue and more muscular tissue than other non-coronary arteries. The thickness of the media ranges from 150 to 350 μm (average 200 μm) made up of several layers of smooth muscle cells helically oriented. The media layer is separated from the adventitia layer by the external elastic membrane, which consists of an interrupted layer of elastin that is considerably thinner than the internal elastic membrane.

The *adventitia* is the outermost layer and is made up of a network of collagen fibers, elastin fibers, and cells (mainly fibroblasts) enveloped in an amorph tissue containing hydrophilic macromolecules (glycosaminoglycans, proteoglycans, and glycoproteins). The collagen fibers are orientated in the direction of the long axis of the vessel. This network is believed to protect the vessel from over-stretching. The adventitia is surrounded by the vasa-vasorum, which supply the media layer. The thickness of the adventitia ranges from 300 to 500 μm.

Coronary Veins

The basic system of coronary venous anatomy was described several centuries ago. Nevertheless, until the 1990s the cardiology community mainly ignored the anatomy of coronary veins and coronary sinus. One probable reason for this is that the only imaging technique available at the time was the ICA, which usually visualizes the coronary arteries and not the coronary venous system (which needs a specific retrograde angiogram made by injecting contrast into the coronary sinus for visualization); another reason is that, contrary to coronary arteries, there is no notion that atherosclerosis of veins may result in specific coronary venous pathology requiring medical, surgical, or percutaneous treatments. Thus, for many cardiologists, the coronary venous system was, at best, only a distant reminder of their early medical schooldays. Starting from about two decades, however, the venous system was back in vogue and knowledge of its anatomy became relevant. Today, in fact, anatomy of the coronary venous system is essential especially because these venous vessels are used extensively by invasive electrophysiologists for biventricular pacing and ablation of epicardial cardiac arrhythmias, by interventional cardiologists for implanting devices to reduce mitral regurgitation and refractory angina, and by cardiac surgeons for retrograde perfusion during interventions.

From an anatomical point of view, the coronary veins can be subdivided into three systems. The major amount of de-oxygenated blood from the left ventricle is collected by the coronary sinus, which enters the right atrium. A second venous system made up of smaller veins collects the de-oxygenated blood of the right ventricle. These either drain individually into the right atrium or join the right coronary vein to enter directly into the right atrium. In about 20% of cases, however, the right coronary vein drains into the coronary sinus. Finally, a third system is made up of the Thebesian veins, small veins that drain different portions of all cardiac chambers, mainly the right atrium and right ventricle, and end directly and individually in these chambers through unvalved Thebesian orifices.

As general statement it can be said that the left coronary venous system resembles a sponge with multiple interconnected subepicardial tributaries penetrating all myocardial layers. However, the main ramifications of the left coronary venous system are pretty constant and parallel the course of the corresponding coronary arteries. For example, the de-oxygenated blood from the anterior wall of the left ventricle and the anterior half of the interventricular septum are drained by branches of the anterior interventricular vein (also known as the great cardiac vein), which travels side-by-side with the LAD. This vein runs to the left side or the right side of LAD. In some cases, two great cardiac veins are present, one sited on each side of the LAD. Posterior-lateral and anterior-lateral veins drain the de-oxygenated blood back from the lateral wall of the left ventricle, while the middle cardiac vein travels along the posterior interventricular groove, side-by-side with the PDA. Atrial musculature is drained into the coronary sinus by small atrial veins (among these, there is the oblique vein of Marshall, a remnant of the left superior vena cava).

The distribution of the coronary veins may have clinical implications. For example, retrograde cardioplegic myocardial protection through the coronary sinus is an effective method to protect left myocardium, particularly during valvular and coronary interventions. Indeed, it has the advantage of a uniform distribution of the cardioplegic solution. However, owing to the anatomy of coronary veins, retrograde cardioplegia protects only the left ventricle in the majority of patients. The anterior regions of the right ventricle that are not connected to the coronary sinus remain endangered, though some studies suggest that the RV is equally protected whether retrograde or anterograde cardioplegia is used. On the other hand, with anterograde cardioplegia through the aorta, the left ventricle may have nonuniform cooling due to coronary stenoses. A technique for delivery of both retrograde and anterograde cardioplegia simultaneously may be useful.

CT volume rendering modality is probably the best method to depict the entire coronary sinus and its tributaries (Fig. 7.23). The recent introduction of percutaneous coronary sinus annuloplasty has drawn attention to the ana-

tomical relationship between coronary sinus and mitral annulus. Several percutaneous devices have been introduced in the attempt to reproduce the beneficial effects of surgical annuloplasty by taking advantage of the "supposed" proximity of the coronary sinus to the hinge-line of mitral leaflets. The devices were, in fact, specifically designed for cinching the mitral annulus, with the intent to improve leaflet coaptation and reduce mitral insufficiency. There are two main concerns regarding this percutaneous procedure: first, the percutaneous coronary sinus annuloplasty has been conceived based on the traditional description of the anatomy of coronary sinus, which is believed to travel in the atrioventricular groove very close to the hinge-line of the leaflet. However, this relationship is not always the case. Noninvasive imaging techniques have, in fact, unequivocally demonstrated that in a significant percentage of patients the coronary sinus is located 1–1.5 cm above the mitral annulus adjacent to the atrial wall. In such a case, the device placed into the coronary sinus may cause a traction on the atrial wall instead of the mitral hinge-line, with little or no impact on mitral insufficiency (Figs. 7.23d and 7.24). Second, in a significant percent of patients, branches of LCx course underneath the great cardiac vein and may be damaged by the device.

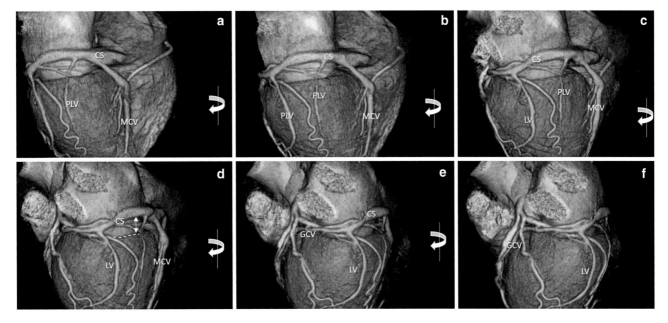

Fig. 7.23 (a–f) CT volume-rendering images showing the coronary sinus (CS), the middle cardiac vein (MCV), the posterior-lateral (PLV) and lateral (LV) veins, and the great cardiac vein (GCV). The volumetric data set is rotated from right-to-left around the y-axis (curved arrow). In panel (d) the doubled-head arrow marks the distance between CS and hinge-line of mitral leaflets (dotted line). See text

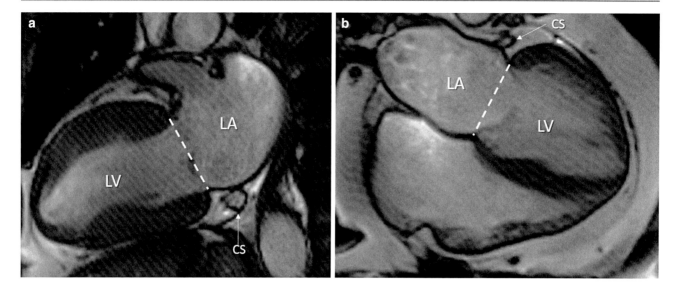

Fig. 7.24 CMR in (**a**) two-chamber and (**b**) four-chamber views. Images clearly show that the coronary sinus (CS) is above the hinge-line of the mitral valve (dotted line). *LA* left atrium, *LV* left ventricle

Suggested Reading

Alexander RW, Griffith GC. Anomalies of the coronary arteries and their clinical significance. Circulation. 1956;14:800–5.

Anderson HV, Shaw RE, Brindis RG, McKay CR, Klein LW, Krone RJ, et al. Risk-adjusted mortality analysis of percutaneous coronary interventions by American College of Cardiology/American Heart Association guidelines recommendations. Am J Cardiol. 2007;99(2):189–96.

Bonetti PO, Lerman LO, Lerman A. Endothelial dysfunction: a marker of atherosclerotic risk. Arterioscler Thromb Vasc Biol. 2003;23(2):168–75.

Loukas M, Groat C, Khangura R, Owens DG, Anderson RH. The normal and abnormal anatomy of the coronary arteries. Clin Anat. 2009;22:114–28.

Picano E, Vañó E, Rehani MM, Cuocolo A, Mont L, Bodi V, et al. The appropriate and justified use of medical radiation in cardiovascular imaging: a position document of the ESC Associations of Cardiovascular Imaging, Percutaneous Cardiovascular Interventions and Electrophysiology. Eur Heart J. 2014;35(10):665–72.

von Lüdinghausen MV. The clinical anatomy of coronary arteries. Adv Anat Embryol Cell Biol. 2003;167:III–VIII, 1–111.

von Lüdinghausen M. Clinical anatomy of cardiac veins, Vv. cardiacae. Surg Radiol Anat. 1987;9:159–68.

Index

© Springer Nature Switzerland AG 2020
F. F. Faletra et al. (eds.), *Atlas of Non-Invasive Imaging in Cardiac Anatomy*, https://doi.org/10.1007/978-3-030-35506-7